MW01170080

(un)expecting

a candid reflection on my journey into motherhood and the
unspoken + unforeseen truths encountered along the way

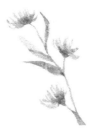

kylee frederick

Ten | 16
PRESS

www.ten16press.com - Waukesha, WI

For information, please contact:

www.ten16press.com
Waukesha, WI

Editor: Lauren Blue
Cover Illustrator: Grace Krause
Cover Designer: Jayden Shambeau
Art Director: Kaeley Dunteman

to c + a:

the one who changed my world,

and the one who walked me through it

contents

the introduction   1

one: let me tell you   8

two: pregnancy   21

three: birth   47

four: home   70

five: feelings   80

six: work   89

the after   101

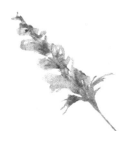

introduction

Let me assure you that I have no idea what I'm doing. I am no expert. I have no authority to be telling you what to expect. The truth is, though, that no one can teach you about YOUR baby. We are all unprepared for the reality of motherhood. We think we're ready because we've read copious amounts of literature. We've all ravished Google with late-night searches for every possible thing that could go wrong (or right). We have experience with kids, or we lack experience but love children (or the idea of children), so we've got this. We have all the stuff. Right? Truth?

The real truth is that none of that really matters.

I generally like to spend my life in a state of, what I consider to be, realistic optimism. I believe wholeheartedly in the power of optimism and positivity, but I also like to keep that in check so I don't float too far from the ground. The perfect combination (for me, not for all of you, I'm sure). So I was optimistic. How hard can it REALLY be? Sure, I know I'll lose some sleep, and I know they'll cry. Those are real facts, yes, but I failed to understand them. I knew them, but I didn't know to have anyone walk

1

me through the comprehension portion of the test. I failed that. The reality was lost on me. Optimism isn't a bad thing to be left with, but yeesh.

When you get home with this tiny human, you may find that your research has served you well and what you had prepared does, indeed, agree with your babe. You may also find that absolutely ZERO of the things you had planned are going to fly. And you're on your own (well, you're not, but it feels like it) to figure out this person that you've created. You may have made them and carried them and planned for them, but believe me when I say that they don't care. They have little personalities and big opinions of their own before they even come out (you can't plan that either), and now you get to decode them like complex hieroglyphs, all while you deal with rediscovering yourself amidst extreme postpartum emotions. What a treat.

This small human (or "these small humans" to you incredible mamas of multiples) that you've created is (are) undoubtedly going to rock your whole world. You won't even recognize it at first. Take heart. The crazy that you feel will bloom into something so beautiful, if you'll just let it.

This is my book of truths uncovered. I'm confident that there will be more. There is no magical point at which everything suddenly makes sense. Whether you've found yourself expecting or just need to remind yourself of how far you've come, this book is about the journey. The devastatingly beautiful journey into motherhood.

As I write these particular words, it is exactly one year from the day that I found out we were expecting. One year. 366 days (leap year). One year is all that it took to alter my entire universe. That's it. As a child, one year seemed to drag on FOREVER. Nothing could come soon enough or fast enough. Double digits . . . first job . . . driver's license . . . graduation. Somehow, though, here I find myself sitting a year later wondering where on earth the time went. Because instead of sitting at work, answering emails and socializing too much with my friends (coworkers, of course), I'm sitting at home, watching my almost four-month-old nap on the baby monitor, and tearing up at the magnitude of his existence. And it all started with a little line on a stick that you pee on. Fairy-tale beginnings for sure.

It was any other day. A Wednesday. I got up, begrudgingly, for work and made my way into the bathroom. We had an event that day that I needed to attend, so my usual easy uniform was out and I needed to put some effort into my appearance. The sun was coming in the window (not supposed to be poetic, just a fact). It was the Wednesday I would normally start my period. My husband had semi-jokingly asked me the day before if I was pregnant. I'm sure it had something to do with my mood. Midweek Kylee was already tired. Work was ramping up for the summer, and I wasn't particularly excited about the event planned for Wednesday. I laughed. But that question stuck in my head. I had bought a few tests a while back after having stopped my birth control, just to have on hand (or in the event that I actually thought I might be pregnant), and decided, "What the heck. Let's waste one."

And then it was positive.

So I took another one because surely I was tired and doing it wrong.

And then it was positive.

The stick said that I was pregnant. Twice, at that.

It didn't really hit me then. I remember my mind kind of swirling and then wondering if I should text my husband. I decided to wait. I wanted to take a few more tests. I thought that maybe I would cry, but I didn't. So I finished getting ready for work, worried about my outfit making me look pregnant, and went on with my day. I made a conscious decision that I was going to be my most normal self and keep this hypothesis to myself. On the way in, I stopped to get more tests. A different brand this time, just to be safe. I took two at work before doing anything else and decided to save the last one for at home again that night.

Positive.

Positive.

I gave myself a pep talk. I needed to be prepared before I started that ten-foot walk from the bathroom to my office. Whether the pee sticks were true or not, I did not want anyone at work being the first to be clued into my situation. Said pee sticks were returned to their packages, wrapped, and shoved down to the very bottom of my bag. Once I opened that office door, it was game on. My work friends would know I was here—and one friend in particular. She could read me like a book. A large-print book at that. I needed to be as normal as possible. Thankfully, I'm not super normal to begin with, but I wasn't taking any chances.

The event that I'd been apathetically waiting to come and be done with ended up serving as a delightful distraction. Not for me, but for everyone else, to distract any attention away from me. The event, and the work day, came and went without suspicion.

Phew.

I drove home just like any other day. My mind was going a million miles a minute, and yet, somehow, there were really no coherent thoughts. Just prayers and colors all swirled together, painting a terrified picture of what I can only describe as timid, fearful joy.

What if it wasn't true? My life could never be the same.

What if it *was* true? My life would never be the same.

I got home before my husband. That was a relief in itself, because I didn't have thoughts—and I especially didn't have words. I let the dogs out, faced myself in the mirror, then took my last test.

THE test.

Positive.

After convincing myself that five positive tests probably weren't wrong (combined with the fact that my period still hadn't started, despite my bringing supplies to work "just in case"), I figured it was probably time to tell my husband. There was some debate because I had so many ideas of cute ways to tell him, but that meant waiting. And I kind of have this thing where I HAVE to tell him everything, because he's my person.

So I approached him casually and asked if he remembered asking me if I was pregnant (yesterday).

"Yes." Stare.

All I could muster in return was a little "I think I might be," followed by a shorter version of the rendition of my day that you just experienced. In all honesty, it still took a while to sink in after that. We were parents? We were expecting?

Expecting. What a word. The dictionary has a lot of definitions that are situation-dependent, but I would expect (hah) that this particular definition is why we use it the way we do during pregnancy: to "believe that (someone or something) will arrive soon." IT SOUNDS SO SIMPLE. And at first, it is. I was expecting that, if everything went how it needed to, a little human would arrive in nine months. Easy peasy.

Even as the appointments begin and you buy your first outfit and think about names . . . simple. Easy. Even as you start thinking about who to tell first, and when, and scouring the internet for the cutest and most original way to tell them . . . simple. Easy. Even as you watch your body change and begin preparing to house an extra human and researching as if parenting were an exam . . . more complicated, but simple. Easy.

The truth is that none of it is easy. Appointments can bring as much anxiety as they do anticipation.

Outfits are adorable but make you worry that you may never get to use them, or that you'll be disappointed by whether you have a little girl or a little boy to fill them.

Names are permanent associations that you have the privilege of attaching to your babe for the REST OF THEIR LIVES. No pressure.

Announcements make this tiny human REAL, and that can be terrifying for a multitude of reasons.

Body change is miraculous and beautiful but can also make

you feel like, while you're doing this incredible thing, you're losing sight of who you are as an individual (and some of the side effects really are just no fun, let's be real).

The prospect of parenting and all that goes along with it . . . well, that one just speaks for itself. Have you ever heard someone say that parenting is easy?

So, while many things are fun and exciting and easier than others, none of it is easy. And those that I talked about? By no means are they the only things. There is so much more. Everyone will find their tailored set of anxieties and insecurities waiting for them on the other side of expecting (and for some, even before that line says yes). If you have a partner in all of this, they'll have their own set of things that you'll be a part of navigating, too. And then you'll have shared anxieties that may make you question what in the world you're doing.

My husband and I had been married almost eight years when I found out that I was pregnant. And no, it wasn't some huge surprise. That's a long time of it just being the two of us (plus the fur babies). That's a long time to get used to doing things a certain way. That's a long time to have a theoretical child that doesn't affect your life, so when a real one comes along, everything that you ever dreamed or hoped comes to fruition. But everything that you ever feared or stressed over also comes to fruition. That's a lot of room for insecurities surrounding change and what that change will look like. So, if you are feeling everything and simultaneously don't know what you're feeling, I get it.

It's not an easy road, no matter the circumstances. Take heart that you're not alone. It's dark under the earth before we bloom.

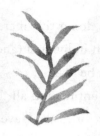

one : let me tell you

Let's start with the things other people tell you.

People are so helpful when they know you're expecting, or at least they try to be. I genuinely believe that for most people, their "advice" comes out of the goodness of their heart or from excitement that they just cannot contain. There's nothing wrong with being helpful . . . if it's helpful. There's nothing wrong with sharing life experiences . . . if it serves a purpose and isn't just offered to project feelings brought forth by nostalgia and a longing for yesterday. There's a difference. Most people don't quite get that, but they'll advise you anyhow. By the time they're done, you will know how every generation before you did diapers, feedings, and sleeping routines, and you'll also know WHY each generation's way of doing it was particularly spectacular, along with how things "are so different now than when I had kids." Be gracious. Be gracious, but also be willing to stand up for yourself. Some people don't know what boundaries are and that they (should) exist. Be willing to teach them. You will be thankful that you did.

None of this is to say that what others tell you is useless, wrong, or absurd. Some of it I have found to be true. Some has been helpful. Some I had forgotten but, upon experiencing it firsthand, returned to me in a beneficial manner. Remember that when you're smiling at someone who is telling you their seventh story about how THESE diapers are better than THOSE diapers and how Dr. Doctor (who is not an actual doctor) has all of the best solutions for everything from diaper rash to language development. Did you know they recommend that brand too? Because they do.

Just You Wait

This was a big one for me. Once people knew that we were expecting, it seemed as though there was ALWAYS a "just you wait" comment. Most were more frustrating or stress-inducing than helpful, although I'm not confident that these are ever meant to be helpful. They remind me more of a reminiscent statement, the speaker looking back on times where they experienced something similar. Or, perhaps, the speaker looking forward in some weird way to seeing just how you'll handle that very circumstance (usually not a positive one) . . .

. . . sitting in church trying to listen to the pastor over the top of a screaming child as their parent sheepishly carries them out of the sanctuary. I feel eyes and look over to see a smirk, followed by a whispered, "*Just you wait.*"

. . . in a public place (store, park, anywhere really) minding my own business and enjoying my freedom when you hear a child screaming and watch them fall to the ground, flailing, while their parent makes an effort to maintain composure in public. I feel eyes and look over to see a smirk, followed by a whispered, "*Just you wait.*"

. . . at an event making small talk when someone starts a story about how their seventy-six-week-old child took their diaper off during their nap and painted a poo masterpiece on the wall of the nursery. I laugh with the others but feel eyes and see a sympathetic smirk, followed by a whispered, "*Just you wait.*"

NOT helpful. I am not waiting for these. Right now, I'd really like to just be able to figure out a schedule where I can pee and not have to go again at the next store, am I right?

But people don't realize this. Honestly, we probably all do it in one way or another, not necessarily regarding pregnancy or motherhood, but about life. We like to forewarn others about the painful realities that we've experienced. Some of it is helpful, yes. Some of it is selfish (come on, admit it) because you know that at some point your younger sibling is going to realize what you've been talking about all along and tell you that you were right about that one thing you've been arguing for your entire lives. You were right, and now they know, and it's such a great feeling. That's where we go with some advice, right? I'm sure that's where other people are going with theirs when they say "Just you wait" to someone who's expecting, but I don't think that expectant mothers are arguing anything. I wasn't. Chances are, I'm not going to call you in two years and say, "Wow, you were right, toddlerhood is ROUGH, and it's no fun cleaning poo off the wall." Chances are, I'll just need a listening ear and some genuine, real support. I think that's how the advice-giving can become ill-received.

Or at least it was for me. I was scared enough; I didn't need people telling me to wait for these horrible things. Sure, I knew I could handle them, but I really just wanted them to verbalize some faith in me instead.

When the Next One Comes

This one still gets me. It bewilders me. I was experiencing my first pregnancy, expecting my first child, and people were making offhand comments about *when the next one comes*. What if I don't want another one? What if I can't have another one? WHAT IF I JUST WANT TO GET TO THE POINT OF ACTUALLY HAVING THIS ONE and then see how we're doing? How about that?

As with most of the other things that people told me, I really don't think anyone meant harm by this particular statement. Every single thing is exacerbated while you're pregnant because you're growing another human, and that's hard work. Not only is your body working hard, but your mind and your heart are running in overdrive, trying to figure out what in the world is happening and how they're allowed to cope with it in an appropriate manner. Give yourself a little grace. Actually, give yourself a lot of grace. Be willing to give it to others as well. Grudges are no good for us, so don't let your babe feel that. No good. There are bigger and better things to worry about between the million things already circling your brain than what your parent's friend's cousin's sister meant when she said not to get rid of anything because then you'll be ready *when the next one comes*. Like, for example, getting ready for *this one*, thank you very much.

Sleep Now While You Can

I definitely did. I am a sleep connoisseur. Well, WAS. Love the stuff. At the time, I was, ironically, sleeping like a baby. Sure, it got uncomfortable toward the end and I had to literally roll myself out of bed, but it never seemed too bad. I wasn't dragging myself through life. I definitely didn't have the respect for it that I do now, though.

You see, people are so quick to tell you to *sleep now*, but they don't tell you why exactly. Yes, we know it's because there is a small child waking you frequently, but they fail to leave out the details. They're also quick to make it sound as though you will never sleep again. That also isn't true. You will. I can't tell you when or for how long, but your baby will sleep, and you will sleep. Eventually.

It would irk me when people told me to *sleep now* because it seemed like this child was an impending doom. Not only am I stressing over every little detail before this babe comes, but now I'm worrying about stockpiling sleep, which isn't really even a thing. It would be an incredible feat of nature if it were possible, but lo, it is not. So, sleep when you can, but don't stress about it because then the stress of thinking about not sleeping in the future will rob you of your sleep joy *now*.

I think I understand where these people are coming from, though. It's like they say—you never know a good thing 'til it's gone. While a baby won't destroy sleep forever (hopefully), it will take you by surprise how much you really do need it. And as much as you love staring at that tiny, little face, you will wish that their eyes would close at some point so that yours could, too. Perhaps it's another of those things that comes across as a warning but is really meant out of self-reflection. Like they would have told their younger selves the same thing, if they could. Or, perhaps it is what it seems and they're secretly gloating inside about how they've regained their sleep but you're about to lose yours. Regardless, DO sleep now, but don't lose sleep over losing sleep that may or may not end up being lost.

Who Will Your Baby Be?

Almost as soon as you find out that you're expecting, people will ask these questions (even people you don't really know that well and may not feel like sharing the answers with, even if you have them): *Do you know what you're having? Are you going to find out? Do you have a name?* Okay. Let's just chill for a minute, Linda.

It seemed as though people were constantly asking these of us. I get it—everyone is curious. Everyone wants to know WHO this little person residing inside your tummy is. I sure wanted to know. But hadn't they ever heard that curiosity bespeaks annoyance (oh, that's not how it goes . . .)? And, more importantly, had it occurred to them that perhaps we didn't want to share that information with just anyone? Maybe we wanted that to be special information that we planned to share with the people who would actually be close with the baby. Maybe we didn't need the whole world to know everything about us, or about this little babe. That's how we felt, at least, and it seemed like others had their own opinions about that on its own. Many people feel entitled to this information, for whatever reason(if they don't, they act like they do). It's refreshing each time you encounter someone who, upon you not answering those questions (especially names), applauds you for keeping it to yourself.

If you're like me and you don't care to put all of your business under the world's microscope, know that it is OKAY to keep things private. This is YOUR pregnancy. Your baby. Your journey. The world will be involved when and how you want them to be, and that is your choice. If this isn't you and you want to shout it from the rooftops, more power to you. There's room for all of us (and let's be honest, your sharing makes people think that I will, which is annoying, but also takes some of the pressure off of me, because you WILL, so thank you!).

Regardless of whether or not you share that information, you will undoubtedly get opinions and predictions. Everyone has a guess as to whether you're having a boy or a girl. People will even argue about it. I'm not sure how we produce these premonitions, but once you're expecting, they come out in full force. It doesn't seem to matter that a 271-5 prediction that it will be a boy won't make your baby a boy. Not only do you have zero control over that, the rest of the world definitely doesn't. But they'll have opinions out the wazoo about it. They'll also ask numerous questions about what symptoms you're experiencing in hopes of better confirming their suspicions. There are SO many old wives' tales about which symptoms accompany which gender . . . . and can I just put it out there that just because you have morning sickness does not mean that you're having a girl? Just because you have heartburn doesn't mean that your babe is going to be a Wookiee. You, my friend, are GROWING a little human inside of you, and your body is going to react however it well pleases. Don't let superstition encroach on your experience.

Last note on gender, something that I didn't realize was a thing, but it is: People may actually go through a pros/cons list with you about boys vs. girls. They might actually make lists. By the end, you'll know every great and beautiful thing there is about having each gender for your child (and also the things that will keep you up even more at night, but we don't need to talk about that—they will). Be ready.

When you do or don't disclose the name(s) that you're considering, also be ready for an onslaught of opinions. This one can get really personal, especially if you have a longstanding tradition of using family names. I can't speak from experience with those, but I'm going to take the chance and say that, even if your family does have a tradition, it is still your choice. This is your human. You are going to raise them. They are going to have this name (theoretically) for their whole life. If you don't want them to be the seventh junior, that has to be okay. If you don't want to utilize a different family member's name in their memory, that has to be okay. It is no person's choice but yours.

I've known a lot of people who, while expecting, have started brainstorming names with close family or friends. More often than not, it seems as though this leads to frustration and hurt feelings. If you have your heart set on a name, don't be afraid to keep it to yourself. Once they see that little face, arguing about their name will (or should) be the last thing on their minds.

We didn't have a name picked for a really long time, but even before we did, we made a decision that we weren't going to share even the contending names with anyone. We wanted it to be our decision, and we wanted it to be special for when our baby arrived. It was worth the hassle of people asking and guessing. We were able to have fun with it, too, and would often refer to him as random names that people knew we would never use. Don't let it be a drag. Names are great, especially when you can finally put a name to that cute little squish face for the first time. YOUR little squish face.

This is the Best

This just is what it is. People will give you their opinions on EVERYTHING, no matter what. It's not exclusive to pregnancy, just exacerbated during, so lookout. You're about to hear THE right way to do everything and THE right products to buy, from everyone, except almost everything that they tell you will be different from what the last person told you. Good luck deciphering the truth in that. Or, more importantly, hear them but create your own opinions. Just because something worked for someone that you happen to know doesn't mean that you must try it or that it will work for you and your little one.

To be fair, motherhood is arguably entirely trial and error, so you will probably have to try multiple things for multiple purposes, but let them be your decisions. Trust those opinions you would normally take to heart. Do your research. Go with your gut. It shouldn't offend anyone if you don't use the same bassinet that your coworker's sister had success with, or if you don't opt for the same bottle that your cousin's sister-in-law swears by. Prepare for feeling unreasonably sheepish if you don't use them and have to relay that information to whomever it came recommended by. There's no reason to feel guilty, but you probably will because that person's emotion will be written all over their face. Stay strong. It's not their baby. It's yours. Your journey. You decide.

Opinions of HOW to do things get complicated. Not only do people speak to you from their own experiences, but they do so with gusto. If they've found a way of doing things that has worked miracles for them, they *want* to tell you about it because it probably changed their life. Many of these are worth noting, but it is SO, so important to not get lost in others' ways. You are going to be your own type of mama (and not the type that you anticipate), and you are going to have to figure things out for yourself. Just because it worked for Janet to put her baby down at regimented nap times with a pacifier and a cleverly named swaddle doesn't mean that it will work for you or that you need to try it that way. Just because Lauren swears by walking counterclockwise around the house while singing "Bohemian Rhapsody" to calm her babe doesn't mean that it will work for you (that one probably won't) or that you need to try to do it that way.

The blessing and the burden of first-time motherhood is that we have NO IDEA what we're doing. All of that experience we have babysitting? Doesn't matter. All of that time we spent researching HOW to do things the right way so as not to mess up this fragile young life? Helpful, but it doesn't take into consideration YOUR baby. This is not the baby that the article was modeled after. This is not Kelsey's baby. This is not Ashley's baby. This is YOUR baby. This is your opportunity to do things your own way that is perfect and special for you. Don't let other people ruin that experience and pressure you to do things a certain way (their way). Embrace the gift that you have of really getting to know your sweet little babe, even when you're left wishing that it was as simple as counterclockwise walking to "Bohemian Rhapsody."

You Will Never Be the Same

These words, or some variation of them, came out of at least half of the people who found out I was expecting. They seem harmless enough, honest. And I can see why—I would imagine that, yes, you will never be the same after having a child. Your body changes. Your schedule changes. Your relationships change. Your whole world changes. So yes, this is one that I believed and even understood. I did not, however, comprehend the PROFOUND truth that hides inside these six words. Read them carefully.

YOU

WILL

NEVER

BE

THE

SAME.

You will never be the same. Ever. Never ever.

Let me break it down for you. "You" references, well, YOU. You as a person. You as a spouse, as a daughter, as a friend . . . as a character in your own life.

"Will" foreshadows the future. Future tense. A state of being. You ARE pregnant (present). You WILL never be the same (future). The state of who you are is not going to be familiar to you.

NEVER. Not in a lifetime, not in a million years.

To "be," as in a state of existence. As in your state of existence.

The same. "Same" means to be like another. In fact, it is defined as meaning to be *identical; not different.* Identical. On its own, "same" would indicate that you do not change. You remain YOU: the person that you are today, with all of the quirks and perks that go along with that. The words before, "you will never be," indicate that sameness is not possible. In fact, it is quite impossible.

So, I repeat (as so many did to me): you will never be the same.

Let that sink in for a minute.

Sit in it.

Relish in it.

Let it scare you a little bit, because it should.

Our inability to maintain sameness with the person that we are prior to giving birth is terrifying. We have gone our entire lives trying to be a person that we enjoy and are proud to be. Maybe we've even overcome some huge obstacles to be the person that we are today. Maybe we're struggling right now with knowing who we are in this very moment. Maybe we don't like who we are. That (all of us—the good, the bad, the insecure, the exuberant) all becomes the foundation for the new you that is born with your child. It doesn't happen overnight, but the process starts in the blink of an eye. Motherhood is challenging. It is trying. It is exhausting. It is exceptionally joy-filled, if we let it be, and it changes us.

I knew in my head that they were right when they said this. I thought that I knew what I was getting into. The truth is . . . you can't. We'll get into it more later, but there is absolutely no way for you to prepare yourself for the change that happens as soon as that babe is earth-side. You will never, ever, ever be the same. And oh, how sweet it is.

....

I want to preface the rest of this book by reminding you that this is just me telling my own experience. Even then, it is only my experience so far (as I write this, I'm only four months in, but I'm out of that "fourth trimester" that they so lovingly refer to). In no way am I saying that you WILL go through the same things, or that you SHOULD. In fact, I would anticipate that most of you will have some of these same experiences but that you'll also have some that are unique to you. Embrace that. Pregnancy, birth, and motherhood are no joke. They are no small feat. Do not discredit yourself. Do not minimize what you are going through, because it is incredible. It is incredibly difficult and challenging. It will change you as a person. It is one of the most beautiful things. And you have the privilege of embracing it.

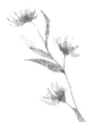

two : pregnancy

The world wasn't as magical as I thought it might be once I found out I was pregnant. You see, I was anticipating this great revelation, some sort of cosmic shift that would blaze the trail for my pregnancy journey into motherhood. That didn't happen. There was no sparkle. The sun wasn't shining extra bright. If I'm being honest, my first two reactions to that extra little line were fear and anxiety. Happiness was there, but it was guarded. It was cautious. There were SO many things that could go wrong, and I thought through all of them, immediately.

I might not actually be pregnant. These tests might all be wrong. Hormones are crazy. I haven't even had any symptoms. What if something happens? What if this was a big mistake? What if it's not just ONE? I can't tell anyone, but I want to tell everyone. I don't want to tell anyone because it might not be for real. It might not last. Do I actually want this? I wonder what they'll be like. Did they just kick? Can I feel that? Who are you, little person? Little person. A BABY. I don't know how to be a mom. A MOM.

This was too much to process before 8:00 a.m. . . . so I didn't. I sat on it. There was no absolute proof here (okay, sure).

I went about my normal routine, which suddenly felt disrupted. Of all days, I had that lunch to attend, so I couldn't just throw on the usual uniform and feel adequate. Hair was done. Pencil skirt came out, which I immediately questioned (Am I showing already?). Fed the dogs. Didn't leave enough time to eat breakfast before I had to go, so I grabbed something to crumb all over my little car with. Drove to work, thinking of all the ways that I could avoid open, honest conversations with my best work friends throughout the day. Drove to work, thinking of all the ways that I could tell my husband. Drove to work, thinking of all the ways that my life was going to change. Drove to work, praying that if this was all true, that I would be enough.

Despite the fact that I would be right on time as it were, I decided that I needed to stop at the store to get more tests. Maybe the ones I had were from a faulty batch. You never know. People get false readings all the time. I knew I wouldn't be able to focus on anything otherwise, so I detoured from work to the store. Bought a different brand, just to be safe, paranoid that someone I knew was going to be around every corner. Actually drove to work, unsure of anything, but I really had to pee. Convenient.

These tests were happening as soon as I put my things down. I snuck into the bathroom, literally around the corner from my office door (which is at the end of a hallway . . . there really was no sneaking required, but it felt completely necessary).

Positive.

And then the next test.

A very fast positive.

I fought the urge to take the other test and opted to wait until

I got home (you know, in case anything changed between now and then). It was starting to get a little real. What if this was actually true? I wasn't sure how I was going to make it through my day normally, or without telling someone. I'm a notably horrible liar.

Somehow I made it through my day. I was able to sneak out a little earlier than normal after we were done with the event, thus avoiding the typical afternoon chats. Said goodbye to no one. Tucked my tests deep down into my bag for my twenty-foot journey out of the building. Sat in my car, staring into space and thinking about everything all at the same time. Drove home, thinking about the blank test in my bag. Drove home, thinking of all the ways that I could tell my husband. Drove home, thinking of all the ways that my life was going to change. Drove home, praying that if this was all true, that I would be enough.

For some reason, this last test held more significance than the others. It was THE test. This was the one that would tell me. I was going to have this moment with my eyes closed while I waited for the test to decide so that in my brain of memories, there would be a momentous occasion.

I texted my husband, like normal, to let him know that I'd made it home safely (and to see what kind of a timeline I was working with). I greeted the dogs, like normal, and let them both outside. While I waited, I looked around our home, wondering if it would actually house a little person nine months from now. What would that look like? What would that mean? Oh my goodness. OH MY GOODNESS. Mini panic.

Once the dogs were back in the house, I locked myself in

the bathroom with my test. You know, because there were so many people in my empty house to walk in on me.

I got everything laid out and forced myself to close my eyes for the whole two minutes while I waited for the test to be "done." To be done deciding whether or not my life was about to change forever. To be done dictating what the next moments of my life would be like. I prayed for the ability to handle whatever was about to happen or, rather, what was possibly already happening within me.

When I opened my eyes, my timer was past two minutes, and I allowed my eyes to shift to the test.

And then I blinked, just to be sure.

POSITIVE.

It was positive.

I was positive?

I cried a little. I'm not sure what I was crying out of—excitement, or fear, or a myriad of other emotions that were most definitely surging—but I allowed myself to feel that. I needed to, because it still wasn't real. I had always imagined that if and when I was ever pregnant that it would be how you see it in all of the social media posts. Immediate elation. Jovial celebration. Cute pictures to store away until I was ready to share them. I wasn't ready for any of that. Don't get me wrong—I WAS happy. It just wasn't the moment that had existed in my imagination. I suppose not many things in life are, but this one felt different.

My husband wasn't home yet, so I sat on the floor for a while just thinking about the immensity of it all. A baby. OUR baby. Inside of me. Existing. Living. Growing.

Apparently I had never *really* thought about pregnancy, because as I sat there pondering, I decided that it was one of those untouchable subjects. I have a few close friends with whom I have sporadic conversations about things that are just TOO much to comprehend. Space is one. Heaven. The ocean. Pregnancy is my fourth. HOW is it possible? HOW? A living, BREATHING human existing inside of another person. I just can't.

Husband. He would be home soon. In that moment, it was decided that waiting to tell him wasn't really an option, for a few reasons. As noted, I'm a horrible liar. Sometimes I actually feel incapable of lying because it makes me sick to my stomach. I apologized once at work for retaliating during a prank war (a mutual activity). Aye. Secondly, I wasn't about to try and wait for something in the mail to tell him for me. And, let's be real. He knew that I was supposed to start my lady business soon.

So . . . I approached him casually after he'd been home for a little bit. He was in the kitchen, looking for something in the fridge. Instead of feeling jubilant excitement, I was nervous. My stomach was in knots, and I could feel the tears balling up in my throat on their way to spilling out. I didn't know if he would be happy. I definitely knew that he wouldn't be expecting the words that were about to come out of my mouth. I definitely knew that he wouldn't be expecting me to alter the projection of our life together with less than twenty words.

I asked if he remembered asking me if I was pregnant (yesterday). After a yes and a stare, all I could muster was a little

"I think I'm pregnant," followed by a shorter version of the rendition of my day that you just experienced.

It was liberating to not hold in anymore but terrifying to finally acknowledge what had been floating around in my mind and heart and body all day.

We hugged.

There was a lot of emotion in that hug. A lot of insecurity and apprehensiveness. A lot of hope.

In all honesty, it still took a while to sink in after that. It wasn't a Hallmark moment. It wasn't a cute rom-com scene. It was just real life, and it was hard to process. It was scary and exciting and almost a little absurd.

In one moment, we were parents. We were expecting.

Expecting.

Never in a million years are you prepared to know exactly what you're expecting. I still don't know what to expect, and I'm four months in at this point. Obviously, you're expecting a baby (perhaps even more than one). What you don't bargain for is everything that comes with it. I'm not talking about the oodles of baby clothes and toys and books and diapers and wipes and products and, oh my goodness, all the things (you don't think that there will be, but trust me—you're about to have a BUNCH of stuff). I'm talking about the emotions—the raw, world-altering emotions that you'll experience. I'm talking about the perspective that you'll gain—you will never look at anything in life the same ever again. I'm talking about the fear and anxiety that will become so profound. I'm talking about this sweet, little babe that takes up ALL of the space inside of you in every regard. Your body. Your mind. Your heart and soul. And that's only the tip of the iceberg. Expect all of those things, and so much more.

Expecting.

It took a little while for this to really sink in. I can't speak for my husband, but it took me longer than I ever would have dreamed just to believe that I actually was pregnant. I didn't expect to feel that way. I thought that it would immediately become my reality. I'd start all of the things that lead up to the baby. I'd start to show. Rainbows and sparkles would follow me wherever I'd go. But really . . . none of that was how it went. We decided early on that we weren't going to tell ANYONE for quite some time. I think that we were both nervous. There were so many unknowns . . . so many things that could go wrong (we're both overthinkers, so I knew this would be fun) . . . so many things to consider before bringing other people into it. AND, really, I could still go to my first appointment and find out that there wasn't actually a little human inside of me. Crazier things have happened.

I didn't really know what to do next. When I called my primary care doctor, they asked which ob-gyn I wanted to be referred to. In my naivety, I hadn't even thought about that. I didn't know that I was supposed to think about that! All I knew was that I wanted a female doctor (nothing against the guys—just not for me). There was a doctor that a few friends from work had used recently and raved about, so I threw her name out there. Thankfully, she was accepting patients, so my doctor's office referred me and pretty much said, "Congrats, good luck, we'll talk to you once you're done there." This was on a Wednesday.

So . . . I waited. I hadn't heard anything by Friday (I'm impatient), so I called the OB office to see if there was something that I needed to do. The lady on the line handled me with grace, which I needed. She confirmed that they had received the referral but indicated that it would need to go under review before they scheduled anything. She couldn't give me a day. She could give me a timeframe of days (that *s* there means plural, as in multiple)—and this is aside from the impending weekend, where we all know those things won't happen. I thanked her and set about with my worrying and uncertainty (and maybe a tiny bit of dreaming about who this little person would be, if they did indeed exist).

I despise timeframes. They leave so much unknown. So much time for nothing and for everything. Not knowing anything for sure but definitely feeling everything. Not having anything planned but definitely in the process of making plans for the rest of my life. Days.

I waited. For a reason that escapes me, I had a day off of work that following week. As I was wandering aimlessly around a store, my phone started ringing. I almost ignored it because I didn't recognize the number, but I picked up at the last minute. It was FINALLY them. They had confirmed my referral, and I was officially a patient. In my brain, I was expecting them to want to see me like right now, but they were annoyingly calm (in the moment, it was hard to remember that they literally do this for a job and, while pregnancy is exciting, my particular pregnancy was not exploding their world like it was mine). We scheduled an appointment for the next week, and I played it off at work as a regular doctor's appointment that got approved without question. Phew.

More waiting. When the day finally came, I didn't know how I was going to cover my tracks. A good friend at work was naturally curious and asked way too many questions about the nature of my appointment. Under normal circumstances, I would have happily obliged, but this time I had to both curb my excitement *and* tell her truths that didn't give anything away but would still appease (yes, I'm this bad at lying). Somehow I made it out of there without her, or anyone else, the wiser. When I got to my car, I remember just sitting there for a minute. I was itching to go, but I was also about to hear whether or not my life was going to change completely. The enormity of that moment did not escape me.

The appointment itself was extremely anticlimactic. When I got there, I had to do a urine test, which made sense but also surprised me that they didn't want more proof than that. A few minutes after, someone came to meet me in a cubicle and verified that I was, indeed, pregnant. Expecting. She gave me a folder full of information about the office and what to expect. I couldn't have known then, but now, gosh, there was so much that the folder didn't have. I was given the rundown of how appointments would work, and we scheduled my next: the first ultrasound. With a congratulatory smile from the nurse, I was off, left with all of this information to process and try and regurgitate back to my husband. It seems so simple. It didn't feel simple. None of it felt simple.

I was actually pregnant.

There was a little babe growing inside of me.

A terrifying little miracle.

I was overwhelmed by it all. We were going to have a baby.

Scratch that. We HAD a baby. Already. They were little, but they were there. The enormity of that revelation took me a while to digest. We were parents. How on earth were we going to be parents?

In the time between appointments, I tried to convince myself that I was pregnant (which was difficult because I was trying to be normal to every other person on earth). We had officially decided that we didn't want to tell anyone until close to the end of the first trimester. You never realize how great of people you have in your life until they're constantly checking in on you when you *don't* want them to.

[Side note: These people are your people. Love them fiercely. They will also be the ones who show up for you and love you even when you don't know what you need after you've had your little babe.]

Thankfully, I didn't have many symptoms. My prenatal vitamins gave me some nausea, but I learned to take them with orange juice, which helped. My hair had been falling out in copious amounts for a few weeks, so that continued for a while. I hadn't realized that was possible—everyone always talks about getting more luscious hair while they're pregnant. It's a thing, though—my doctor confirmed it. And mine fell out like crazy, especially at first. Not my favorite development, but it was better than a lot of the side effects that I've heard people talk about. Despite the fact that I felt like I was showing, I was not. It was definitely all in my head. That was handy, though, for the secret keeping.

Symptoms are peculiar things. I thought going into it that I was going to be one hundred percent MISERABLE one hundred percent of the time. It was going to be like one of the plagues had hit me. I was going to be endlessly tired, endlessly hungry, and endlessly moody. I was going to have random food cravings that didn't make sense, and I was going to have luscious locks of hair, and I was going to have cankles. And I was going to forget EVERYTHING—because mom brain. And that's just how it was going to be. But NONE of that was true. Not even a little bit.

I felt normal. A little nauseous every now and then, and a little more tired than usual, but otherwise normal. Happy. A little more anxious. That's a lie. A lot more anxious. But more of a happy anxious, like anticipation mixed with apprehension. It was confusing and mesmerizing all at the same time. Part of it was probably founded in the fact that I STILL didn't fully believe it. I didn't know if I would be able to until I was staring that little babe in the face.

The only person that I told was my close friend at work. I wanted someone in the office to know in case anything were to happen while I was there, and she's one of my people, so it just made sense. I almost couldn't do it. It was the end of the day. I'd waited to make sure that everyone else had left so that there was no chance of accidental eavesdropping. Based on the doctor's estimation, I was exactly eight weeks along. There had been a million ways I thought of telling her, but I was so nervous that I could barely breathe, nonetheless think.

Like I often did, I peeked into her doorway before I left. She was sitting at her desk, working on something that she probably wasn't very excited about. I lingered for an awkward amount of time, working up the courage to say ANYTHING.

And then I told her that I knew it was a ways out, but wondered if she had plans in January because I might need help with something.

What?

I may have said something else, but that's the best that I remember. And now I just have to laugh thinking about it, because it was a ridiculous thing to say.

It took her a solid thirty seconds before she realized what I was saying. And then she started crying. And then I started crying. The first time I'd *really* cried since we found out. I didn't realize how much I needed to until that moment.

Telling her broke something in me. All of the fear and excitement and apprehension that had been pent up inside of me for so long—it was validated. Speaking those words brought this baby to life in a way that I didn't know needed to happen. In the thirty seconds that it took her to understand my nervous gibberish, all of those things rose up. And, for the first time, I allowed myself to actually FEEL all of them. It was not at all how I thought that conversation was going to go, but it was exactly what it needed to be.

We cried, we laughed at my nervousness, and she was sworn to secrecy.

The next morning, I came in to a sweet little gift hiding under my desk, from her of course. The teeniest little animal-printed moccasins, a book, and a card that spoke confidence and hope into me. Her excitement was catching.

Time seemed to creep at a dramatically slow pace as we waited for ultrasound day to come. Work was picking up for both my husband and me, so we had a lot of distractions. They weren't very effective, but they were distractions nonetheless. I was in la-la land most of the time and was busy trying to pick out my own pair of moccasin booties. Did it matter that they were aqua? For some reason it REALLY mattered that they were a shade of blue. It was bothering me. I didn't think that I wanted a boy. I had always pictured myself with a little girl. It actually wasn't even an option in my mind, to have a boy, even though I tried to remind myself to be (optimistically) realistic. I bought them anyhow.

Then it finally came. It was ultrasound day. I'd managed to schedule the appointment for a day that we both had off, during our little anniversary getaway. A sweet little gift to ourselves. The appointment was in the morning, so I spent time getting ready and then spent the rest of my time frantically worrying about when I could last pee before leaving and how much water I would need to drink on our five-minute drive in order to still have a full bladder by the time we got there. The logistics were killer. It had to be perfect. They told me to have a full bladder, so it had to be full. I kept chugging water the whole way there and had to pee by the time we were seated, so I figured I had done it right.

Everything seemed so surreal. It was just a plain, little room, dimly lit. The ultrasound tech had a kind face and demeanor that matched. She had me lie back and my husband sit in a chair facing the monitor as she gently explained the process. Squirt the jelly. Find the baby with the wand. Take the picture. A simple process, sure, but the MOST complicated outcome. This was the moment where everything was going to become real. I was so hopeful, but so terrified.

And then there it was. Right there, on the screen.

A little gummy bear shadow, dancing around its cozy cave.

My little gummy bear. Our little gummy bear.

Our baby.

IT WAS ACTUALLY THERE.

Everything looked as it should. The baby was healthy, as far as could be told. They were growing appropriately to what their estimated gestation was. This was happening, and everything was OKAY. Even though I wasn't fully convinced of this "being pregnant" thing, I desperately needed to know that everything was okay. All of my initial fears went out the window. I knew they would return, because we were barely nine weeks along and a lot could happen, but for now, everything was okay. This little person was okay. That in itself was a blessing.

We left with ultrasound pictures in tow. I held them ever so carefully so that they wouldn't crease. I didn't ever want to forget this moment.

I can't say that things immediately changed after that for me. It wasn't like some magical moment where the stars aligned and suddenly everything was completely real. I was still apprehensive, but there was proof enough for me to start thinking of this little being less as a possibility and more as a *them*. My them. Little gummy bear baby.

And I loved them. I just couldn't possibly know how much.

After the appointment, we waited some more. We still weren't ready to tell anyone else. It was kind of a fun little (BIG) secret to keep. As time went on, the not telling became our normal, and just thinking about telling everyone became harder. I wasn't expecting that. At first, I was SO excited to tell everyone, picturing their faces when they found out that we, of all people, were going to have a baby. But over time, that excitement transformed into anxiety. I started to get nervous about sharing our secret. I liked having this little person to ourselves. I didn't want to share them. These feelings took me by surprise.

Close to a month after that first ultrasound, we began seriously deliberating when and how to tell our families. I made gift purchases (because for some reason it makes sense to buy things for other people just to tell them that you're having a baby) and plotted how these conversations would go. Over the course of the next month, we shared our news, strategically, with our families and closest friends, but asked them to keep it quiet until we were ready for the general public to know. After each conversation, I remember thinking that it was much more anticlimactic than I had expected. There it was again, a reality-crushing expectation. There were some tears. Everyone voiced their excitement. So many hugs. Lots of questions.

But no sparkle. No magic. No dancing in my womb.

I actually felt some anxiety afterward. Not because of anything said or done—our people were so incredibly supportive and encouraging—and I can't exactly place where it came from. I was feeling particularly possessive. Possessive of this baby. Possessive of this experience. Possessive of the time between now and their arrival. And I was still feeling apprehensive. That's a difficult thing to be feeling when you're trying to be jubilant.

We decided to not do a social media announcement. We wanted to tell the people we were close to in person, individually, and our families and close friends were gracious enough to not share the news with other people until we were ready. There didn't seem to be any benefit to posting a cute picture online (even though I had some prepared) for the whole world to see if those who we cared about already knew. It wasn't about them. It was about us. For the first time in my life, I felt okay being selfish. It felt good to believe it. It was about us.

We weren't scheduled to have another ultrasound until the physiology one where we could (WOULD) find out whether this was a little girl or a little boy. My appointments in between were really just check-ins with my doctor to test proteins and sugars and listen to babe's heartbeat. We found out that I had become mildly anemic (that can be a thing—the babes can steal your iron, apparently). I was actually the lowest weight I'd been in over a year. Any nausea that had been there was gone. I bought a pregnancy pillow to cuddle with at night to try and train myself to stop sleeping on my stomach early, so that when the time came that I couldn't anymore, there might be some hope. I had a streak of eating ramen every day for lunch for quite a long time. My husband and I created a shared note for names but didn't put much effort into it yet; it seemed wasteful to get set on a name just to find out that they were the opposite gender. I started a nursery collage. This was life.

Most days I still felt like I was just living out a story. Who's to say that the heartbeat wasn't just a recording attached to the wand that they used to find it? Who's to say that there was actually a little human growing inside of me (despite the fact that I was ACTUALLY starting to see little changes in my belly now)? It was all so surreal, and I wondered if I would ever get to a point of true acceptance.

It wasn't for lack of *want*. Of course the baby was wanted. They were already loved, as much as you can love something that you don't quite fully understand. I just felt oddly disconnected. When I started to really ask myself why, I realized that I was protecting myself. I was scared. I was scared that it was too good to be true, that things were going too well. I was scared that something was going to happen to the baby. So, if I just distanced myself, I would save myself some heartache. I would save myself the pain of loss. I KNEW that this wasn't true; I would experience devastating loss and heartache even if I pretended not to be attached. These things were inevitable in that situation.

A lot of days were spent within these thoughts. Willing myself to not feel, and willing myself to feel. Because whether everything went right or everything went wrong, I would regret not cherishing every single moment that I had been given with this babe.

Over time, the word got out and I would receive random congratulations. There were a few comments about how they must have missed the announcement and how they had heard from so-and-so's aunt's work friend (my point exactly). People would ask if we had found out the gender. People would ask if we were going to find out. People would tell me what it was going to be. People would ask if we had a name. This is when a lot of those helpful things that people *did* tell me came out. Yay.

The majority of people were Team Girl. My first-informed good friend, however, was 2697% Team Boy from the very moment that I told her. I always joked that if it was a boy, I was going to blame her for his entire life. My answer to everyone was that I was partial to a girl but ultimately just wanted the babe to be healthy. That wasn't a lie. All I wanted was for them to continue to be okay. To have all of whatever parts they had. Ever since the first ultrasound, though, I'd had a feeling. An inkling. A little spark poking at my heart and soul. And I never shared it with anyone because I didn't know if I was ready for it to be true.

Then, so quickly, it was the night before the day. THE DAY. The day where one little word was going to change everything. Everything would be defined. We were going to have a daughter. We were going to have a son. I don't think that I slept well, or much. Most of my night was spent praying for an open mind and an open heart. That healthy was enough. I felt guilty for even having to pray for those things. I shouldn't have to, right? But I did. I had to. I had to be okay before I went. Had to be prepared for whatever the day brought.

I was shaking by the time I got to the doctor's office. The anticipation, the nerves, the apprehension . . . it was all coming to the surface. The worst part was feeling ashamed for feeling that way. Like I was doing a disservice to this little person inside. It wasn't their fault, or their choice. What I had expected to be a whimsical, magical appointment had quickly become daunting. My husband met me at the doctor's from work, and we walked in together from the parking lot. I briefly toyed with the idea of *not* finding out, but that really wasn't an option. I couldn't handle not knowing. (Honestly, I don't know how anyone does —my control issues? Perhaps.)

This ultrasound tech wasn't nearly as personable as our first. She didn't have much to say the entire time, and I couldn't even see the screen for part of the show. Talk about not living up to expectations. This wasn't going how I thought it would. Everyone should be as excited to find out the gender of our baby, right? Even this person who doesn't know us and who might not even normally work here because the offices share staff. In my head, sure. She should definitely be excited.

When she spoke, I didn't even realize what was happening at first.

"It looks like it's a boy."

That's all she said. Quietly, at that. As if it were just an afterthought to whisperingly mention. As if it weren't something that may or may not change the entire trajectory of everything that I had been wondering and hoping and dreaming for.

That's it.

Twenty-one weeks of waiting and wondering, this great mystery of life, concluded in about two seconds. IT'S A BOY. World-altering.

And then she moved on.

I did my best to keep up with the few things that she said the rest of the time. They had to perform a secondary internal ultrasound to get a better view of the positioning of the placenta; she didn't seem worried, but that sounded like a big deal to me. I wouldn't know more until the doctor reviewed the ultrasound images. Even better.

I left feeling nervous.

Sad.

Unsure.

Emotional.

Frustrated that I felt all of these things when I should only be ecstatic.

We had originally planned to do a balloon reveal that evening. Part of the family was headed out for over a week on vacation the next day, so we thought it would be a fun send-off. Instead, I got home and asked our family if I could bring them surprise cupcakes in lieu of a get-together, using tiredness as my main reason for ditching the event idea. I assumed that they would read into it as me needing time, which was true, and thankfully they obliged.

Having that settled, I went to the bathroom and cried. I gave myself a few minutes, then came out to finish the cupcakes that I had started the day before. They just needed the filling colored accordingly.

Blue.

They needed blue filling.

Baby blue.

Baby boy.

We were having a baby boy.

I must have looked as lost as I felt, because my husband hugged me and asked if I was okay. I immediately started crying again. We stood like that for a while, in the kitchen, in front of the unfinished filling.

People don't talk about gender disappointment like they should. I feel horrible even typing that word—*disappointment*—but it's so significant. And because people don't talk about it, I think it makes it worse. I know I felt worse. I didn't *not* want a boy. I had always just pictured a girl. And I didn't know how to explain that to people. I felt like I was mourning the loss of something that I'd never had to begin with. I didn't know how to mourn it, especially because it hurt to think that mourning was necessary. It was so necessary, though.

In order to move forward with the joy and excitement that was warranted, I needed to let go of those expectations. I needed to let go of the things that I had planned, even though I shouldn't have planned them to begin with. I needed to embrace the fact that a part of me knew this was a little boy from the very beginning, and perhaps that's why I had had such a difficult time facing myself so far.

In that moment, crying, I decided to move forward. It wasn't without hesitation. It didn't fashion immediate healing. But it was what needed to happen. I had a little boy.

My little boy.

I was this little boy's mama, and he deserved every bit of me.

Wiping my face, I pulled robin's-egg blue food coloring out of my baking supplies and finished the filling. Blue. We took a picture to commemorate, tongues covered in that blue frosting. Tired smiles. Hopeful hearts.

Everyone was so excited. Those who knew me best checked to see how I was doing with the news. I loved them for it, but it also made me feel guilty all over again. I really was excited; I just needed time. Healing happens over time.

It's funny how the tune changes once people know what you're having. Suddenly, even the people who voted girls over boys were saying how great boys are. How fun they are. How special it would be to have a mama's boy. The more I thought about it, I knew how right they were, and it soothed me. I thought about a whole new myriad of opportunities that we would have with a boy. I thought about my husband having a little mini-me running around. Going fishing. Learning about cars. I thought about what kind of man he might be when he grew up. I'd loved this baby all along, but it was more personal now. Over a shorter time than I expected, I stopped mourning the loss of the dream of a girl and fell in love with this little boy. Our little boy.

Time really started to move quickly once we knew. It felt like overnight we were over halfway through the pregnancy, even though time had CRAWLED leading up to the gender ultrasound. We didn't have a name. I hadn't really started on the nursery yet. All of a sudden, there were SO many things to do. The registry had to be finished. Showers had to be planned. Who do you want to attend? Who do you need to appease by having attend? Circumcising, or no? Birth plan? Are we having visitors? When are we having visitors? Posting on social media? It was a never-ending barrage of questions, questions that I hadn't thought all that much about.

Not so simple, despite our efforts. It had seemed simple. Have the baby. Love them. Live happily ever after.

Not too long after, the showers started. I was exceptionally nervous. All of these people just wanted to love and support us, which is such an incredible gift on its own. I despise being the center of attention even under normal circumstances, and these were far from normal (whether or not it was true, it felt very much like people had been just waiting for this baby, and now it was HAPPENING). I didn't want people asking me questions that I wasn't prepared to answer. I didn't want people telling me "helpful" things that I knew were just going to add to my anxiety. I was nervous that we would get a lot of random stuff that we didn't want, and I felt guilty for feeling that way about all of those things.

I started to realize that I was good at that.

Feeling guilty.

What I couldn't seem to figure out was WHY.

Why I felt guilty. Why I felt guilty about feeling that way.

I never was able to figure it out. I went through all of the conversations and planning and showers feeling thankful, but anxious. Protective.

And then I realized that I didn't want to share him.

The prospect of being pregnant had me excited to go through all of these things, almost like they were my rites of passage into motherhood.

Announcements.

Showers.

Celebrations.

The reality of being pregnant and having kept him a secret for so long was making me extra protective and possessive. I wanted to keep him just to myself for a while longer, but that wasn't really an option anymore.

Everyone was SO excited to celebrate him. To celebrate us. It was overwhelming.

My whole life, I have hated being the center of attention, for any reason. Public speaking gives me horrible anxiety. Once in high school, I had to recite "To be or not to be" (the whole thing) in front of class. I pretty much blocked out the entire memory. I passed, but I'm not sure if it was because my teacher felt bad for me or if I actually did it. We'll never know. But, you get my gist. That's how it is. I hate the limelight. Why on earth had I decided to do something that would put me directly in the middle of everything and everyone?

Oye.

I learned to suck it up, and I learned more than ever that the people in my life who love me love me HARD. They loved this little boy just as hard. Possibly more. It was such an incredibly beautiful thing. All I had to do was be present, truly present, and say thank you.

Time continued to fly by. All my life I'd heard people talk about how time goes by faster as you get older. Surely that couldn't be a thing.

Oh, it is.

Halloween came and went. I dressed up for work as Pooh Bear, tummy full of my little honey.

Thanksgiving.

Christmas.

With each holiday, it became more real. Not because I almost couldn't see my toes anymore or because of the drumming in my belly that happened most evenings. But because I realized that these were the last holidays my husband and I would celebrate our normal way. The next year it would be us + him. It would be we. Our little family.

The reality of that was hard to swallow. As I thought about all of the things that we were doing together for the "last" time, anxiety started to creep in again.

EIGHTEEN YEARS.

That's our minimum commitment to growing and raising this little human.

Were we really ready for this? Were we cut out to be parents? Were we going to be upset by the way he would change our lives?

We didn't know anything else.

We didn't KNOW anything.

Looking back, I was a fool. My anxiety was properly placed at the time, but gosh. I was wrong. He makes everything BETTER. [I still find myself missing the days of it just being my husband and me, but now it's hard to imagine life without our boy. I'm excited for the holidays as they come because we get to bear witness to his experiences. We get to facilitate those. We get to see his face light up with absolute JOY at the smallest things. It's everything that I could never have expected.]

We crept closer and closer to my due date. Friends at work were rallying for labor to start there, so that they would know when it was happening.

I was secretly hoping that he would be born a day early: my dad's birthday. I had an appointment with my doctor that day, and I spent the morning daydreaming about being in labor and not knowing about it, being ushered right over to the hospital, and having him that day. Happy Birthday, Papa. I wasn't feeling anything, but a girl can dream, right? I didn't know what to expect to be feeling anyhow—every expectation was a figment of my imagination at this point. I constantly thought about it but also couldn't think about it too much because I would freak myself out if I did.

Fear of giving birth was so real for me. How?

HOW?

It wasn't my day.

My doctor checked, and little to nothing was happening. I told her that I had been crampy for a few days, almost like I felt before my period, and she said that it can be a sign of early labor. I got excited. She followed that up by assuring me that it could also just be my body preparing. Thanks.

We set three more appointments for the upcoming week if he didn't come between now and then. Non-stress test (just the name sounds stressful). Another ultrasound to make sure he wasn't running out of room. Another non-stress test. I was hopeful for a while that I would go into the next week, for another chance to see him via ultrasound. Then I realized that I could actually SEE HIM if he would just come (duh).

I decided I was ready. I didn't know what I was ready for. I didn't know what to expect. I didn't know ANYTHING. But I wanted to meet him.

His due date came and went.

And the next day.

Come on, baby boy.

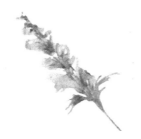

three : birth

It was Saturday.

Two days after his due date. 40 + 2, as they say.

I was relieved to have made it through the work week. As much as I love my work friends, I really didn't want to go into labor there. We were looking forward to a slow, lazy weekend. No plans. No place to be. No agenda.

My husband had been feeling really poorly all week, so I let him sleep in. When he did get up, the morning proved to be worse than the night before. It was going to be a good recovery day. Pancakes. Coffee. R&R.

And then I peed my pants.

Well, I actually didn't know WHAT had happened, but that's what it felt like. Just a little bit. Not out of the question, right? I was not queen over my own bladder at this point.

I slowly came out of the bedroom to my husband, who was sitting on the couch. Not wanting to unnecessarily worry him, I started my sentence with "Not to freak you out, but . . ." (for the record, this is not a calming preface) and then proceeded to tell him what had maybe happened. He, being the rational one, asked if I should call the doctor.

I thought about it. Assessed how I was feeling. How my body was feeling. I didn't FEEL anything. I felt normal. Large, but normal. A little excited, but normal. Suddenly terrified, but normal.

I told him that I would wait and see if it happened again and call if it did.

Again, being the rational one, he suggested that I just call to see what the on-call doctor had to say about it.

I called and explained to the triage nurse what had happened. She asked me some questions and told me that the doctor would follow up. I prepared to continue on with my day.

It was only a matter of minutes before the doctor called me directly. She wanted me at the hospital to check if what had "leaked" was amniotic fluid. For some reason, I was surprised that they could check that. She was going to call ahead to the birthing center to let them know I was coming.

I almost didn't want to tell my husband. I knew he was feeling terrible. This was going to be stressful whether something happened or not. It wasn't what we had planned for the day. But I didn't really have a choice.

He asked if we should bring the bags.

I hadn't even considered the possibility that we might actually go there, stay there, and have this baby.

I decided yes. It was a bit of a trip to the hospital, and it seemed wiser to take them and not need them than to not bring them and need to come back for them. Sensible. I grabbed the checklist that I'd had ready for months now. Suddenly, it was foreign to me. It felt like something that I had never thought

I'd need, but now it was time and I did. Bizarre. The whole thing was bizarre. Surreal.

While my husband grabbed everything, I changed out of my comfy clothes, because . . . society. Why I felt the need to be presentable, I don't know.

And then it happened again.

I had actually just peed, so I knew it wasn't that.

AGH.

I waited to tell him until after we were already in the car.

Our drive to the hospital was about thirty minutes. It was a quiet drive in. I really didn't think that this was it.

I was too calm.

I didn't FEEL anything special.

I wasn't in pain.

I didn't have a magical inkling.

I didn't feel the way that I expected, had I truly been in labor. And it has to feel that way, right?

We got to the hospital and, after peeing (for real) yet again, found our way up to the birthing center. They were expecting us, just like the doctor said they would be.

107.

I knew this room already.

It was the room that I had sat in for five hours, two and a half months before, for observation after a kamikaze deer jumped (I'm not joking) off of a hill and into the side of my car while I was driving.

It was the room that we were shown on our hospital tour at the end of our birthing class.

It doesn't really get more telling than that. I remember looking around that room on the day of our tour, the prospect of giving birth still so fresh and foreign, thinking how weird it was. Weird that that's where babies come into this world. Weird that that's where more strangers than I'd be comfortable with in an elevator would see more parts of me than I was comfortable thinking about.

But this day, it was just a room.

I wasn't freaking out (yet).

The nurse took my information and then asked me to change into a gown. She gave me two, one for the back (for modesty, you know).

They completed a swab test to check the fluid.

We waited.

It felt like an eternity.

I kept looking at my husband, knowing how miserable he felt. And I still didn't feel anything, so . . . I was pretty confident that we were going home to wait some more.

A while later, the on-call doctor came in. She was kind. I had been nervous about not having my own doctor, especially because I still wasn't even comfortable with HER being in my lady business, but I really didn't have a choice here.

She started talking about time and options and plans.

Wait, what?

I asked, because no one had actually said it. "We're staying?"

"YES." She smiled.

I panicked.

Even though I don't feel anything?

50

Even though there was no eventful waterfall?

Even though my husband is actually really ill and right now doesn't feel like the best time?

Even though I'm realizing that I'm not actually prepared for this?

Even though I don't have a "plan," because I thought it was silly to make one?

Even though...

YES.

That was it. One word. A confirmation. We were staying. There was no going home in a few minutes. There was no waiting to see when he'd come.

THIS WAS ACTUALLY HAPPENING.

When we went home, it wouldn't be just us. From this moment on, it was going to be different. Everything was about to change.

The definitiveness of that was terrifying.

Was I excited? Yes. Somewhere in there. Was I everything else? For sure.

This was the last time that we would drive somewhere as a couple, without a baby or a babysitter . . .

The last time I would feel this sweet babe inside of me . . .

The last time he would be safe and sound, tucked away within . . .

This was it. Ready or not.

We took a picture once we knew we were staying. I look back at it often because I want to remember us then. I want to remember all of those beautiful and terrifying things that I was feeling. I want to remember that I existed before my sweet boy was here. I want to remember that moment in time when everything was about to change.

There's a bit of a rush once your water breaks (or leaks, in my case) because your babe is more exposed than before. Ideally, you meet your baby within twenty-four hours of that happening. The only problem was that nothing really was happening.

I had expected such a different experience.

Pain.

Writhing.

Obvious signs.

Noticeable progression.

None of that was true for me. I didn't even feel what the nurses told me that I would be feeling. I never felt contractions like they said I would. They were all lower, like cramps. Not even that bad at first. Actually, not that bad for a long while.

Things weren't moving along like I expected them to. Things weren't moving along like the doctor wanted them to.

Can I say? The checks were the WORST. No part of labor that I had experienced to this point was as painful as them checking to see whether or not I was actually, indeed, progressing.

And what even does that mean, "progressing"? It felt like a bit of an ironic word choice, because nothing felt like it was progressing. To progress means to move forward, onward. Time was standing still. Nurses were visiting, and they were checking, and we were walking, and they were checking, and monitoring, and it was like . . . nothing. Like I was watching everything from outside of my own body.

The hands on the clock kept moving, and things kept happening, but it was still absolutely surreal to me that THIS was happening. That my body was working on expelling this little human. I was just there, waiting.

Waiting to feel what they told me to expect.

Waiting to feel what I had expected to feel.

Waiting to FEEL anything.

I wasn't excited.

I wasn't really nervous.

I wasn't really anything.

I wish that I had been more purposefully present, especially in those first hours. I wish that I had taken time to note everything rather than just being along for the ride. I want to remember every moment that led me to him. Most of it is a blur. Looking back, I don't know that I would've had any other choice than that, but I do wish that I had more to recollect.

As things continued to NOT progress, despite our countless trips up and down the hallways, they started rattling off options. As if I had any idea of what I was doing.

They decided to give me something to help "ripen" everything, supposedly encouraging more active labor.

I remember that word specifically because it made me want to giggle like a schoolgirl (literally—one time in high school, my best friend and I had to do a presentation on both reproductive systems, in front of our older peers, and we were not the most "informed" teenagers). But that's beside the point.

I can't say whether or not anything "ripened," but I can

say that they were happy with the results. I could barely tell a difference, despite that. I still felt crampy. Period-ish. Nothing earth-shattering. None of the "split from stem to stern" terror that I had heard about.

It didn't feel like he was doing a "coming home" dance inside. Or sliding down the rainbow to life. Or anything magical like that.

My poor husband was exhausted. Still felt like poo. I tried to not bother him because, for whatever reason, I was more concerned about him than I was about being in labor.

Go figure.

After a while longer, they decided that they were going to induce because things weren't moving along as quickly as they would have liked.

Thanks to the little holes in his roof, little babe needed to get out sooner rather than later. Cue my first time feeling completely helpless—before he even came out. What better foreshadowing to parenthood?

Saturday was disappearing. It was late evening, somehow.

After the induction, the contractions forced me to pay more attention to them. They were still crampy. EXTREMELY crampy, actually, but in more of a take-your-breath-away way.

Going into this, I had no plan. No birth plan. No magical mood-setting paraphernalia. I was going to wing it. I knew that I really didn't want an epidural, but mostly because I was terrified of it.

I wish that I'd thought about it a little bit more.

As things got harder to work through, I started to give up a little. I was tired. We'd been there for almost twelve hours already.

I tried to just breathe through the contractions but found myself holding my breath for most of them instead.

My husband lovingly reminded me that I didn't need to prove anything to anyone. That I had a choice and was allowed to make it. He granted me that permission, and I am thankful for it.

It took a little while, but eventually I gave in. I'm not sure exactly what I gave in to, but that's what it felt like.

Giving in.

Giving up.

Caving.

I decided to get the epidural.

I was terrified.

Needle.

Spine.

Those two words really don't voluntarily belong in a sentence together.

The anesthesiologist came in not too long after I had made my decision.

It wasn't pleasant.

His first attempt didn't take, so the moments that I spent trying to hunch over just so, while having contractions, had to be repeated.

It hurt.

The physical hurt didn't last long. Once his second attempt took and was in place, things started calming down. A weird sensation, for sure.

I didn't really experience tightening anymore. My legs were

super heavy, like I was walking through syrup mixed with pillow stuffing. I couldn't feel anything but pressure when they checked me again (HALLELUJAH).

It hurt me inside to do it, though. That lasted longer than the needle pokes. Still hurts, if we're being honest. Despite having my husband's support (not that we were pushing one way or the other, but sometimes I just need that validation in my life), I felt like I had let someone down.

Like a quitter.

Like I had failed my very first task as a mama, and our boy wasn't even here yet.

Looking back, I'm thankful that I did it, because his birth story could have ended very differently had I not. We'll get to that, but retrospect is always clearer.

So now I was a little tired, and sad, but things were happening. The nurses turned the lights down and told me to try to get some rest. The doctor came in to check another time and discovered that the little mister was "sunny-side up."

It sounds cheery, right?

Negative.

Simply put, this means that the babe is face-up rather than face-down.

COOL! We get to see their tiny little face first, right?

Nope.

They consider it safer and more ideal for the baby to be face-down for their entrance into the world.

How do you get an unborn baby to spin?

With hands.

And positioning.

And more hands.

And more acrobatics.

This is all fine and dandy, except once you have an epidural, you can't really feel or move your lower half with your own power.

I spent the next couple of hours being turned like a rotisserie chicken and molded like Play-Doh in the hopes that he would change his mind and spin his body. My husband, who originally wanted the very least to do with the functions of childbirth, ended up being my second nurse and helping turn and position me.

Rest was little, for both of us.

At 2:00 a.m., the doctor came in to check again and said that it was time to start getting ready to push.

WHAT?

Oh yeah, we still need to get him out.

The room went from dark, cave-like, and serene to bright and bustling in a matter of minutes.

I remember looking at the time and thinking that within the hour I would be face-to-face with this little guy.

A baby.

Our baby.

It wasn't until 3:00 that everything was actually in place and ready. To "push" is a much more complex verb when in conjunction with labor, FYI. Pushing is a weird thing. It's a complicated action, and it's daunting (for me, at least) because the number of people who have seen your lady parts grows exponentially.

Mortifying, but necessary.

I do wish that I could have felt more, simply because I think that it would have helped me realize that things were actually HAPPENING down there. It was kind of like working out and being exhausted for no reason because you can't actually feel the stress on the lower half of your body.

Odd sensations.

Tiring activity.

They told me that, ideally, I would push when a contraction came because that is the most efficient. Makes sense. Except I couldn't really feel the contractions, so I felt a bit like I was pushing blind.

My nurse was INCREDIBLE. I wish that I knew her last name so that I could find her and tell her how she impacted my life. She didn't give up on me. She wouldn't let me give up. She kept telling me that I was one of the best and strongest pushers she'd ever seen (that's not a compliment that holds much bearing until you're in this situation).

When I first started, they told me that I wouldn't push for longer than two hours because of how taxing it is, especially with a first baby.

Those two hours came and went, and I remember looking at the clock thinking that he would HAVE to come out now because the time had passed.

That's not how it works?

Time to come out, baby boy.

At one point, he had flipped back again, so they were trying to get him to re-flip.

At another point, his head was stuck in my pelvis (just thinking about this makes me so claustrophobic for him), so they tried to use the little suction vacuum. That was a laughable moment (in retrospect, of course). The doctor about fell backward when it slipped off the babe's head and splattered who knows what all over the back of the room.

I was getting SO tired.

I couldn't feel anything.

I didn't have a clue where he was in my body, but they kept saying that they could see him.

It felt like they could see him for a long time.

Around 6:00, I started to panic.

It felt like he was never going to come out, that he was going to be stuck in there.

I was tired.

I was emotional.

Those feelings, especially together, never bode well for me.

My emotional journey through pregnancy can be summed up in one experience, which my family now lovingly refers to as the "getting stuck in a winter coat" feeling. It is exactly how it sounds. Sometime near the end of my pregnancy, I put my winter coat on, and the zipper got stuck just past my large bump. Which meant that even though I was about to go outside, I was stuck. It was hot. I couldn't breathe. I thought maybe I could pull the coat over my head, but panicked further when I realized that my exceptional belly wasn't going to allow me the wiggle room to do so without getting even more stuck. My husband wanted to pull the zipper up to figure out where it was stuck.

Excuse me?

My best option was a pair of scissors. Coats are replaceable, and I surely was going to die in this coat if it didn't come off ASAP.

My logical husband talked me, his crazy-eyed wife, down and got my zipper unstuck.

I didn't zip it again for a long time.

And now, when I feel anxious and panicked and stuck, I'm right back in that moment. Yeah. It felt like that.

Except this time, I couldn't cut the coat off. I couldn't stand outside in the cold to counteract the frantic heat building up inside of me.

They saw it happening. My husband saw it happening.

I was able to ask for a washcloth and fan. It helped, at least for the moment.

I remember wondering how long they were going to make me do this and if a C-section would be easier, even though it wasn't something that I wanted.

I closed my eyes and bore down, trying to will him out because I couldn't actually feel if I was successfully pushing.

And then everyone started yelling at me to LOOK!

He was already out.

HE. WAS. OUT.

HE. WAS. HERE.

My baby was here.

We had done it.

He was here, and he was perfect.

And now I'm crying as I write this because oh my GOSH I had NO IDEA of how life-altering that moment was.

6:35 a.m.

A lot of things ended in that moment, but so much more began.

It was surreal to hold him. I actually couldn't believe that he had somehow come from inside of me. Sometimes I still have a really hard time believing that.

At some point, the rest came out after him, but I didn't feel a thing. I was so enamored.

My husband ended up cutting the cord. We cuddled him before they took him to clean him off and get his measurements.

8 pounds and 20.5 inches of pure love.

Those couple of minutes after he was born are so precious to me. I spent them staring, in love and in such disbelief.

I don't really have words to describe that feeling. I spent my pregnancy not allowing myself to think too deeply into the future, not to think too deeply about what he would be like. I had few expectations. But I can tell you that he surpassed any that I could possibly have had.

He was more than I could have dreamed for. Or prayed for.

More than any little girl.

More than any other little boy.

More than anything else in this world.

He was everything. Everything that I didn't know I wanted, or needed. My missing piece.

Everything about him was perfect. His little nose. All of his little fingers. His belly that fell into sync with mine. His deep, dark eyes that stared straight into my soul. He fit so perfectly, like I'd been pining for him my whole life.

This might be one of the most cliché string of things I've ever said, but it is all breathtakingly TRUE:

Time stopped, and it was love at first sight. Love so different from anything I'd ever encountered. Different from what I'd imagined. Different from what I'd expected.

Deep, soul-filling love. Explosive. Colorful.

My sun, my moon, and all my stars.

And I knew, in that moment, that from now on, I would be a different person. I had no idea what that meant, or what that would come to mean. I had no idea of the implications of my world getting turned upside down, in a good way. No idea of the struggle to come. No idea of the joy to come.

I just knew that he was here. And perfect. Perfectly mine.

Ours. We created this human.

By some miracle, we, even with all of our great imperfections, created this perfect little person.

REALITY, though.

Everything was a whirlwind after that moment. They offered me a shower to clean up, and I remember them being surprised at how easily I was able to stand on my own. I had a shower supervisor, just in case. Despite the fact that an undetermined number of people had just seen some of my most intimate parts and pieces of life, this was still awkward for me.

Can I call it sheer will? I really just wanted to be done and back with my baby. And to sleep. Oh, to sleep. A siren call of the future.

I knew in my head that things were going to happen in

my nethers. I had read books. Seen pictures. Watched videos. Researched, researched, and researched again. I was prepared.

Yet, somehow, when it was actually happening, it didn't even cross my mind to think about what was HAPPENING to my body and what my body was enduring (probably also because I couldn't feel it happening).

WOW. I remember washing up and being ASTOUNDED at the ways my body had changed in the last twenty-four hours. Wow. Just WOW.

I slid into the cloud-soft pajama dress that I'd prepared, and they gave me a fresh pair of rubber-dotted hospital socks. They were tan. Ugly, but emotionally beautiful in that moment. I made sure to tuck the first pair into my bag. There was no part of this experience that I was going to leave behind, regardless of what those socks had seen and suffered.

Despite my insisting that I was just fine and clearly capable of standing, I lowered myself into the wheelchair that they were required to transport me in.

And then they gave me my baby.

Both mildly clean.

Both reeling from the last nineteen hours.

Both exhausted.

My husband joined us.

Also reeling from the last nineteen hours.

Also exhausted.

But here we were. The THREE of us. On our first short but significant journey (down the hall) as a little family.

Room 125.

It wasn't much different from our delivery room. As cozy as a hospital room can get.

We had a few minutes to ourselves after that, and I don't remember my husband and I even talking. Just staring at our baby, staring at each other. I think I asked how he was feeling (I still felt horribly that this all had to happen when he was sick). I remember thinking that I should be crying, but I was too overwhelmed to even do that.

This was it.

This was us now.

We + him.

So beautiful. So profound. So incredibly indescribable.

We decided that we weren't going to wait as long as we thought we would to tell people. I didn't even use the text draft that I had saved in my phone, awaiting the details. I winged it. This was not a draft-fulfilled type of moment.

It was into the morning by the time we were settled in our room, and we soon had all of our immediate family planning to come visit right after church.

We watched some HGTV. Took turns cuddling our baby, our son. Tried to "rest." Talked to multiple medical professionals about insurance and breastfeeding and circumcision and what to expect. Talked to nurses, who were gracious and helpful with everything from helping him latch to helping us learn how to swaddle him like a tightly-wrapped burrito. Talked to a few friends.

Then they were there. Everyone came at almost the same time, which was good. And then a bit overwhelming.

Overwhelming because in the middle of it, I realized that I really just wanted quiet time with my boys.

Overwhelming because of the emotions that having that much LOVE in one room stirred up.

Overwhelming because I was exhausted, in every sense of the word.

Overwhelming because I looked at my son and finally experienced how my parents felt about me.

The next two and a half days were like a slow hurricane. The highlights?

Frequent checks on me and on the baby. Apparently, in order to see that you're recovering properly, that includes pushing firmly on the womb from which you just expelled a child. Repeatedly. Beware.

So much poop talk. I can firmly attest that I have never talked about poop so much in my entire life. My poop. Poop potential. Iron supplements. Stool softeners. His poop. His need to poop before we left. Lots of poop.

Many nurses and other staff members giving so much advice (opinions?). Bless their hearts, they were amazing, but holy wow overwhelming.

Lots of HGTV. *Love It or List It* marathon for what felt like our entire stay.

Desperately wanting sleep but desperately not wanting to let my fresh, new babe out of my sight.

Note here: It was against everything in my instinct to use the nursery. I did not want to use the nursery. It scared me and made me anxious to be away from him. It made me feel like I was already not living up to being the best mama for our boy.

But it was SUCH a blessing, amidst the anxiety. The little sleep that I was able to get was that much more than I would have gotten had I not used it. A friendly reminder for those of you giving birth in a hospital: generally, the staff of the birth center are *pretty* well educated and trained, specifically regarding babies. Especially more than me. So really, aside from me being his mama, he was probably safer with them (you know, alert, educated, and trained professionals) than he was with me for those portions of the first two nights (you know, sleep-deprived, anxious, emotional, irrational new mom).

Desperately wanting to be at home but desperately not wanting to be without the guidance of the swaths of professionals who had been directing us so far.

Contemplating. Staring. Living in a state of continuous amazement.

Amazed at this little boy.

Amazed.

It felt like we were in the hospital for an eternity, but then it was Tuesday and everyone was talking to us about going home and discharge paperwork and follow-up appointments.

We actually had to go HOME? To our house?

To the place in the middle of nowhere where we, as newly pegged parents, were to raise this tiny, fragile, squishy, adorable, incredible bundle of baby boy?

Where there were no doctors or helpful nurses?

Where there was no nursery?

Wait.

Really?

They were serious. It was time.

I felt like I should have been ecstatic. Overjoyed, even. Grateful?

I was scared. This was real life, coming in hot. No amount of years working with kids, or being around other people's kids, had prepared me like I thought that it would.

IT'S NOT THE SAME.

I had a fear of what? I'm not even sure. Everything?

Fear of failing.

Fear of not being enough.

Fear of not being able to live life the way we had before.

Fear of ruining my husband's life.

Fear of this being a mistake.

Fear of letting my son down.

My son.

MY SON.

And then I looked down, and for a second, it all went away, and I was left with this immense love. My heart actually felt like it could explode. I know that's cliché, but I think it almost happened. I have never felt it so full. Ever.

And I told myself that we were going to be okay. It was going to be alright. It had to be. He was counting on me, even though he didn't know it yet.

And I remembered that he was created for me, and I for him. I remembered that because I knew I would forget in the moments when I would need to remember most.

We packed everything up, and I took some pictures to commemorate the space in which we spent our first two and a half days as a family. It felt so trivial to take them. It was a hospital room. With an uncomfortable bed. And an uncomfortable couch. And with walls that had seen too much of my body.

But that room . . .

The first place where my baby slept outside of my body.

Where I learned how to use my body to feed him.

Where I watched my husband snuggle him.

Where I experienced some of the hardest moments of my life to that point.

Where our families and closest friends met him for the first time.

125.

We got the all-clear for our departure, so now it was up to us to work up the courage to leave this safe space.

We got him dressed for the first time in the only outfit that kind of fit him from the four that I couldn't decide between when I was packing our bags.

We struggled with the car seat. It's easy, right? Yeah. Once you know. But we didn't know.

He SCREAMED.

I asked myself why it wasn't okay for me to just carry him all the way home. Nothing could protect him better than me, right?

Don't worry. We used the car seat. But I didn't like it. Neither did he.

I remember looking at my husband before we left the hospital and feeling just about every emotion that I knew could exist. The resounding winners, though?

Hope.

And love.

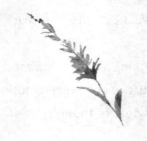

four : home

And then you're home.

Home, to your house.

Home, away from the hospital.

Away from all of the people who actually know what's going on.

Away from all of the people who were helping you survive the first few days.

And then it gets extremely REAL.

There is a BABY.

He is MY baby.

I am not babysitting.

I am not respite care.

I am not living in an alternate reality where I get to see what my future baby looks like and think *Ohmygosh he's so freaking ADORABLE.*

I am just home. In OUR house. With OUR baby. Alone.

My husband was there, of course, doing everything that he could. Had I known better, I would have asked for more. I would have asked for his help to navigate all of this. But I felt like I had to do it on my own. Not because of anything he did or said (quite the opposite—he was so willing to help with anything and everything), but because I didn't know what I needed. How could I expect him to know?

And everything that I thought I knew, or that I had expected, or that I had anticipated . . . it just vanished.

POOF.

Looking back, I know I was heavily hormone-influenced. But there, in that moment, it felt like a blissfully joyful, desolate situation. That's the best way that I can describe it.

We unloaded our things from the car as if we had gotten groceries. Except there was a baby.

Our dogs were waiting for us, like they always did. They didn't have a clue as to what was about to happen. Poor things. We had sent a few receiving blankets home for them, in hopes that it might get them used to his smell. It was a nice effort, but I don't know that it did anything for their attitudes toward him.

We walked in the house, and everything was the same.

Same furniture.

Same things.

Same mess.

But it was like I was seeing it all for the first time.

We put the car seat on the couch so that the dogs could see but not touch. And then I remember thinking, *Okay . . . but what now?*

What do you DO with a newborn?

I could think of a million things that needed to be done.

Cleaning.

Laundry.

Organizing.

Dishes from when we left unexpectedly.

Looking back, I wish that I could tell myself to just
LET IT BE.

I learned that it's not so simple, to just change who you are and what you worry about. Imagine that.

While my husband started putting things away, I settled into the couch with our baby curled up on my belly, sound asleep, almost as if he were still in it. Part of me wished that he was. His change of address really complicated things for everyone.

To be honest with you, I don't remember many of the details or specific moments beyond that. I do know that I was acutely unaware.

In that moment, with him curled up into me, everything felt calm and right, even though I didn't really know what I was doing. Part of me wishes that I could go back and warn myself about what was to come. Part of me doesn't, because I wouldn't have had the journey without the struggle.

So much struggle.

So much heartache.

So much anxiety.

So much joy.

I think my husband and I both felt like we should be DO-ING something. It was difficult to grasp that all we really needed to do in that moment was tend to our babe.

The little dog didn't seem to notice him much. The big baby

of a dog was standoffish, pouty, and jealous. Neither were aggressive at any point, but Mosley, the big baby, definitely seemed to know that his scheduled, quiet existence was about to be disrupted in the biggest way.

[There's not much dog advice that I can offer, just be aware that it may not be the picture-perfect friendship that you imagined when you were pregnant. It took a long time for our big dog to finally start showing interest in our son and to stop being as sulky.]

I honestly don't remember what happened after that. All of the things, and not much at all.

From the moment we got home, I was obsessive about writing everything down. The doctors had freaked me out with all their talk about how soon and how many types of diapers he should be having, making sure that I was alternating sides for nursing, burping him often enough and correctly . . . the list went on.

In the bag of stuff that was sent home with us from the hospital, there was a little booklet that you could use to write down feeding and diaper times, with details for each. That became my lifeline. I wrote every little thing down, and when I didn't have the booklet on-hand, I kept a note in my phone. I still have that long, long note to look back on and remind me of how far we've come. How far I've come (even though, to this day, I still keep a log for him each day, so . . . there's that).

Looking back, I think that I clutched at that so closely because it was one thing that I COULD control. I was learning so quickly that aside from doing the things I needed to do to keep our child alive, most of it was really out of my hands. And, as we'll get to, my emotions were COMPLETELY out of my hands. Keeping this eat/feed/sleep journal was my anchor.

I found myself not wanting any visitors. Not only was I overwhelmed, but instead of wanting to show him off, like I had imagined, I wanted the absolute opposite. All I wanted was to be at home, alone, with my husband and baby. It felt like too much for anything else.

I had to brush that aside, with visitors at the house within a few days of us being home from the hospital. If we could do the coming-home experience again, I would have waited longer for visitors, or constructed the visits differently. I was not in a good spot for that. For conversation. For help, even well-placed. I would tell myself that I had the power to control visits, even if it meant making people wait longer than *they* wanted.

I was tired.

I was anxious.

I was extremely possessive.

These emotions were all really new for me, especially the anxiety. Anyone who knows me would tell you that I'm generally a super laid-back person. Easy-going. Adaptable.

Nope.

And I'm sure it was even more extreme to others, especially to my husband, watching me from the outside. I was so turned around that it took me a while to even realize that what I was experiencing was NORMAL postpartum, but not normal for me. And that's a super critical distinction.

The days were long and yet flew by at warp speed. What days were, I'm not really sure, because time was all its own. Days were nights. Nights were days. Sometimes they were both at the same time.

I didn't realize what I didn't know until I didn't know it. Trying to read about how to care for a baby and get them on a schedule is REALLY HARD when you're trying to care for that same baby and get them on a schedule. But, going into it, I didn't know that it would be like that.

No one told me that I might end up super anal and anxious about EVERY. LITTLE. THING.

That I might feel anxious and moody every evening around 5:00 because I knew that nighttime was coming and that it meant cluster feeding. And a sleepless first half of the night for me. And a sleepless second half of the night for my husband.

That I might harbor negativity toward breastfeeding because it felt like it was consuming my every moment and thought.

That I might supplement with formula because my sweet boy was just SO hungry.

That I might switch exclusively to formula because I couldn't keep up with his feeding and with what scraps of my mental health were still intact.

That I might regret doing that, when all was said and done.

That I can't control everything.

That I might still not be able to sleep, even when he was asleep, because I was worried about him not being okay.

That it's actually impossible to make a small babe follow a

strict schedule, and that I really should just enjoy that precious extra time with him because it's fleeting.

That I might isolate myself from my friends and my family because I could barely handle myself. And that I might not be able to bring myself to explain that to them.

That I might cry all the time.

So many things.

I had to learn to surrender. I had to recognize that I was struggling. HARD. And I had to deal with that.

I reached out to another mama friend after a few weeks and told her what I was going through. I don't know if I just needed to express it, or if I was trying to get her to validate all that I was experiencing. Both happened. And she encouraged me to get in touch with my doctor.

When I reached out to my doctor, I learned that what I was feeling was completely normal. How could it be normal when I felt so out of control? So abnormal?

She wanted me to keep myself in check and follow up with her if nothing changed. Apparently, everything that I was experiencing—the anxiety, the emotions, the whole lot—was likely rooted in my hormonal imbalance after birth.

Wow.

I gave myself the weekend. I REALLY didn't want to go in to see her. I didn't WANT it to be postpartum anxiety, but I also really didn't want to feel this way anymore. It wasn't fair to my husband. It wasn't fair to my little boy. It wasn't fair to me.

I don't know if it was my self-pep talk or a few more days

of giving my body time to regulate itself, but I truly was feeling a little more "normal" by the time the weekend was through. I probably overexaggerated my newfound jubilation to my doctor, but she gave me the go-ahead to just keep monitoring myself, with the expectation to follow up if I started experiencing anything severe again.

This wasn't some miraculous turnaround, I want you to know. I don't think it works like that (or at least it hasn't for me). But it morphs. It changes.

Just like you will.

Just like I have.

Just like I am.

Even after I started to feel more like myself, things were still different. Things were still hard. Babies seem so simple sometimes because they really require little and do little.

DON'T BE FOOLED. They are extremely complex.

Nobody told me that a normal amount of spitting up looks like they're not keeping any of their food down.

That sometimes they spit up explosively, and that can be normal on occasion (seriously, a geyser).

That baby vomit covering three-quarters of my outfit at some point isn't always enough to make me feel the need to change.

That they don't just sleep where I want them to, and that I would have to help him learn to sleep in those places.

That everything I planned to never do would cross my mind as an option once I was worn down from trying the same things over and over again without success.

That I might have to try four different kinds of swaddles before finding one that my baby likes (tolerates).

That I might have a Hulk baby who could break out of almost any swaddle, therefore increasing the anxiety around safe sleep.

That the cute stuff might not work as well as the old-school, practical options (and that the cute REALLY doesn't matter).

That I would discover an entirely new appreciation and love for my husband that cannot be put into words.

That people might judge me for doing things the way that I'm doing them. And people WILL judge me for doing things the way I'm doing them. Yes, I said what I said.

That some people won't.

That people will surprise you.

People surprised me.

With their candor.

Their frankness.

Their patience.

Their tolerance.

Their unwavering support.

Their love.

That you will surprise you. I surprised me. I discovered a whole new person that I didn't know existed. I did not exist the way that I am before my sweet boy. It wasn't possible. And I'm not saying that it's perfect. Holy wow, I am not perfect.

But I've changed, and I am so thankful for it. Thankful for the opportunity to grow, despite the struggle.

Thankful for the challenge and joy that has gotten me here.
Thankful for my babe, who loves me however I am.

Lean into the chaos. If I could go back and tell myself something, it would be this: Fighting and dodging and manipulat-
ing? It's a waste of time. A waste of energy. A waste of precious
moments spent stressing over a nap that didn't run long enough
rather than scooping that babe up and snuggling for an extra ten
minutes. Don't waste time stressing about things that cannot be
controlled. A rhythm will work itself out organically, if you give it
room to. Have grace for expectations. Have grace for frustrations.
Accept the grace that others have for you. Lean in, and fall into a
rhythm of grace.

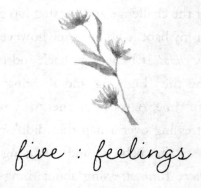

five : feelings

Let me start by telling you this: no matter how in tune you are with your own body and emotions, you have no idea what's coming. I HAD NO IDEA of my true scope of emotions until that postpartum flux. I also had no idea how many emotions a single person can experience in one day, or even within one moment. Moreover, I had ZERO control over the ebb and flow of said emotions. None. No control whatsoever. Even though I could acknowledge what I was feeling, the why would always escape me, and that was (and is) sometimes the worst part because it would make me feel crazy (okay, crazier).

It was terrifying for me.

I have always considered myself to have a higher emotional intelligence. I'm easily able to identify and empathize with others, and I've always been able to easily self-regulate my emotions. Even during pregnancy, this was true. It was more difficult, and there were stronger emotions to regulate, but I never felt *unlike* myself. A little moodier at times, sure, but still myself. Postpartum was a brave new world of emotions, and I did not feel brave. I felt everything but brave. Literally everything.

Enamored.

Exhausted.

Proud.

Mournful.

Overjoyed.

Overwhelmed.

Thankful.

Wrecked.

How on earth could I feel so many different things at once? It seemed like I should only be experiencing positive emotions. Joy that my sweet babe was earth-side. Gratitude that everything went smoothly. Contentment to be home and healthy as a new family. Don't get me wrong, I felt ALL of those things. I already loved that little boy more than I ever imagined I could in a lifetime. But the rest of what I was feeling overshadowed that sometimes, and I didn't understand why. Why I couldn't just be happy all of the time. Why I couldn't just talk myself out of this funk. Why I couldn't understand WHY I felt that way to begin with. We're not talking about five minutes of fleeting weepiness here and there, or crying at a Folgers commercial (let's be real, I did that even before I got pregnant).

One of the more profound moments that stands out in my mind happened during the week that we came home from the hospital (all of those days run together in my mind; there's no way to know what day it was). My husband could tell that I was in need of a break. He took the little one so that I could go shower (hello, new novelty). I was utterly overwhelmed. He could tell that I was overwhelmed, but he didn't know how to help me. I didn't know how he could help me. So I went to shower. I was crying before I even turned the water on. I couldn't understand why. I just felt HEAVY. Broken. Ungrateful. Scared. He came to check on me a few minutes later and found me just standing in the shower, sobbing gut-wrenching soul sobs. He kept assuring me that everything was going to be okay. I kept telling him that I knew. I did. I KNEW it in my brain that everything was going to be okay. We were going to adapt. This little human was going to be incredible. But I couldn't stop.

Part of me didn't want to stop. It was like all of these tears were gushing from the caverns of my soul, and maybe, if I didn't stop—if I just let them come—maybe they would run themselves out. Maybe I could run myself out of emotions so that I could start fresh. Renewed. Maybe I could finally feel like myself again. I couldn't put words to everything that I'd been feeling, but the tears were doing a pretty good job of it. It was devastatingly beautiful, and I allowed myself to feel it all.

That wasn't a stand-alone experience. No one-and-done. The same thing happened multiple times within the first few weeks of being home. I allowed it because I knew that my heart and soul needed it. I needed to be able to feel all of the things that I was feeling, because letting them grow and fester would only result in something unseemly. And I didn't deserve that. My husband didn't deserve that. Our sweet, fresh, new babe didn't deserve that. We all deserved the best version of me that I could muster, despite the undulating emotions that threatened to take me down.

Anything that could be felt, I felt, and I felt it to the extreme. All at once. Over and over again. It shook me to my core, and I hadn't expected any of it. At first, I figured that I was just tired and that my exhausted state had exacerbated high emotions. As the days continued and I continued to FEEL so intensely, I knew that there was more to it.

I was constantly worried about something. Our babe was quite jaundiced for the first few days, so that weighed heavily on my mind and resulted in some unnecessarily stressful internet searches. Was he eating enough? Sleeping enough? Would he ever sleep in his crib? Was I ruining him by letting him nap on me?

It got especially bad in the early evening. Every day, I would feel it come on and start to worry about how the evening and night would go.

Would he cluster feed again?

Would he sleep?

Would I sleep?

Would my husband sleep?

I was wrecked every time. I could immediately feel the difference in myself, and I hated it. I was tense. I was irritable. I was nervous. I was constantly on the verge of sobbing. Not crying. Gut-wrenching sobbing. I felt overwhelmed. I felt like a failure. And this was every single day.

And then every time I would really think about it, I would cry more. How could I be so SELFISH?

So many people want and wait and pray for children. For some it happens, but it takes time. For some it comes by way of another person's child. For some it just becomes a hole in their soul, a dream not come true.

How could I be anything but exceedingly grateful? How could I even formulate the thought of him being anything but EVERYTHING that I didn't know I had needed?

Gosh, what a privilege.

What a blessing.

I was a mess.

I did some research (aka Googling). This is never a good idea, by the way. This is also when I reached out to my friend and told her that I thought I might be struggling with postpartum anxiety. She encouraged me to reach out to my doctor, so I did. In the heat of my emotion that day, I typed up a message to my doctor and told her what I was experiencing.

The intense emotions.

The worry.

The anxiety that flooded my entire being at the same time every day.

I felt a little better as soon as I sent it. It was so validating just to express the way that I was feeling. It wasn't just feeling crazy. It was all emotions. Real, raw emotions.

When the morning came, things didn't seem so hard. I sent a follow-up message letting my doctor know and that I thought maybe I was just going through the hormonal flux of the first few weeks of postpartum. I felt better every morning, though. She asked me to not downplay what I was feeling and reminded me that PPA is very real. She asked me to stay in touch. It was comforting to know that I had someone in my corner.

I struggled hard for another couple of weeks. When I say hard, I mean it. Feelings that had first surfaced after coming home were only exacerbated over time. I was terrified that I had made a mistake. And that was a hard one to swallow. How could I even THINK those words when I loved this baby so much?

I was terrified that things would never be the same.

That I would never have time with my husband again.

That we would never not be stressed.

That we would never not be exhausted.

That he thought we had made a mistake.

That I needed to prevent any frustration from ever happening so that things would never get hard.

That I needed to do everything that I had before.

That I needed to be the same person that I was before.

That I needed to seamlessly make this babe fit into the life that we had established.

I wrecked myself daily over these things. It felt like there was no end in sight. No light at the end of the tunnel. Just a very long, dark, lonely, tearful, exhausting tunnel.

And then, ever so subtle, a flicker. So subtle that it took me a long time to realize it was happening.

I was starting to feel like myself again. It was a different sense of self, but it was refreshing. I was not the same person that I was before having him.

I was gaining confidence as a mama.

I was gaining confidence as a woman.

I was gaining respect for myself.

The nights became less fearsome. The stressors became less encompassing.

I was still terrified. But he was worth it.

He was worth every moment of self-doubt.

Every moment of anxiety.

Every exhausting day.

Every tear.

I shamed myself for ever thinking otherwise. For letting myself FEEL any of those things, and for letting them affect my time with him.

Please don't do this. Don't shame yourself for having emotions. Don't shame yourself for being confused or frustrated or overwhelmed by the fact that you have grown and brought life to a small human and that your life has been IRREVOCABLY changed.

Transformed.

I was transformed.

Every feeling has a purpose.

EVERY.

SINGLE.

PAINFUL.

JOYOUS.

FEELING.

I'm still not the same. Honestly, I doubt I'll ever be the same.

My emotions still get the best of me some days. I'm even more sensitive than when I was before him. I get frustrated at little things easily. I still get anxious sometimes at bedtime when he starts to fuss or if he stirs more than normal in the night. I'm also anxious about other things now. About him being safe. Sleeping well. Eating enough. Sleeping enough. Developing "properly." Worried about when he's too old to want to cuddle. When he's a teenager and I don't know what to do with him. When he moves out of the house. Seriously.

But it's manageable now. I'm not drowning in it like I was.

There are days when I start crying when we rock before I put him down for bed. I can't even tell you why, but the tears come.

They're necessary.

They're beautiful.

They give life to the stirring in my soul that this sweet babe ignites.

I'm overcome. That's the best way I can describe it.

Overcome with joy.

Overcome with uncertainty.

Overcome with all of the emotions I'm learning to home.

Overcome with gratitude.

Overcome with the most immense love for this babe.

My baby.

My little boy.

My miracle.

That's not something they tell you when you're expecting. When you're expecting, people tell you to watch out for those postpartum feelings. They usually say it with an air of humor, as if looking back it were comical, or a fond memory.

Those feelings are no joke.

I have never felt as out of balance and out of control of my life as those first couple of months after having my baby. It was terrifying and exhausting. I was forced to reconcile with my feelings every day. Sometimes more than once a day.

Give room to your emotions. They probably will feel crazy; mine felt crazy. But they're valid. Respect them. Respect what they're trying to accomplish. And talk about them. Talk about them often. Talk about them with people who will lift you up but will also be real with you. People who will cry with you. Talk about them with people you trust. Do not drown yourself in attempting bravery.

If I could go back, I would remind myself that the pressure I felt was placed on me by no one. I did that to myself.

No one expects you to have it all together.

No one expects you to be so brave.

No one expects what you're expecting of yourself.

Be kind to yourself.

Give yourself grace.

Be kind to myself.

Give myself grace.

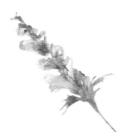

six : work

Work had become a distant thought.

After having our boy, I knew that I was going to eventually have to return to work. That was the arrangement. I never had the desire to be a stay-at-home mom, so it didn't faze me when I was pregnant to think about going back to work. I was expecting to do that. I was expecting that I would be ready to enter back into society and reclaim my position after ten weeks off. That I would be bored. That I would enjoy sharing my time as a professional and as a mama.

As time ticked by, though, I found myself keeping track of the weeks. The first few weeks flew by. Eight weeks left. But that's two whole months, right? No. It's eight weeks. Seven. Six. Five. And then suddenly the countdown transitioned to days because I was within the last month. And instead of preparing myself to return to work, I was freaking out about the prospect of going back. I'd worked in some capacity since I was fourteen. That was my normal. I hadn't thought that my mind would change. We had a plan. A great plan. He would be SO well cared for. And I could go back to working.

But I didn't want to anymore. Every fiber of my being was balking at the thought. How was I supposed to leave this adorable little creation EVERY DAY?

The days kept ticking by. So much anxiety.

I was going to miss all of the milestones.

He was going to forget me.

He was going to grow up thinking that someone else was his mama because he would see them more than me.

I was going to resent my job.

I was going to resent myself for not thinking through the possibility of not going back to work.

I did resent myself for not thinking that through. I still resent myself a little for not thinking that through.

We got to the practice run day of daycare. We had decided it would be best to make it a full day, like an actual work day. I felt annoyed with myself for getting so worked up because it wasn't as if he was staying with strangers. My brother's family was watching him. People that I love. People that I would trust with my own life. His life felt more important.

So I got him ready and dropped him off. I managed to not cry, but it felt like my heart was being ripped out of my chest. I wasted my day shopping for new work clothes. Exhilarating.

It was the most bizarre feeling, being alone. All day, I kept flipping between feeling like the two and a half months prior could have all been a dream and feeling like I was forgetting him in the car, like a piece of me was missing. A piece of me WAS missing. I tried to enjoy my time. I browsed. I wandered. I told myself that this was good for me, and for him. I gave myself a pep talk. Tried to remind myself that this was the plan. This was what I had wanted. It wasn't the most helpful, but it was an effort. I just kept looking at the empty car seat base in the backseat.

I missed him.

I missed his little squish face and his pudgy fingers wrapped around mine.

I missed his smell.

As soon as I could, I headed back to him. I wasn't going to be away for a minute longer than I had to be. And I was concerned. The tiniest part of me was enjoying the freedom of the day, and that scared me. It shouldn't have, because that was a good sign, right? I should be okay with being away from him because I was going to have to be. I should want to have a little time to myself. But I didn't want those things. I felt guilty and sad for even feeling them the teensiest bit.

I pushed those feelings away. I didn't want them. I was used to being with him. I loved being with him. I felt at home when I was with him. I wasn't ready to accept that anything else could be my reality, even though it was inevitable. Because that's what I had wanted. I had been okay with going back to work. And I hadn't been able to come to the conclusion yet that it was okay for me to change my mind. I was allowed to want different things. I was allowed to feel all of those things. And I didn't have to understand them. It was okay just to feel them. To process them. To let them be free to influence me into the person that I had become. The person that I was becoming. The mama that I was becoming.

It was so refreshing to see his face. He was safe. He had been all along. He had done so well, my sister said. He had been HAPPY.

He had been happy without me. That was a lot to swallow.

His happiness wasn't reliant on just me.

For some reason, that was crushing. Heartbreaking.

I wanted only for him to be happy. But I also wanted him to miss me. I wanted him to miss me like I had missed him. In some ways, I wanted to feel justified in my desire to change things so that I could stay home, because he needed me. Right?

I kept telling myself that I should just be thankful. Thankful for an incredible place for him to be while I had to be at work. Thankful for family that loved him so incredulously. Thankful for family that loved me so incredulously. Thankful for the opportunity to work. Thankful for the ability to work. Thankful for a babe who was happy while he was with me and while he was away from me.

But it was hard. It was so hard.

Soul-wrenching hard.

And that was one day. One day away from him.

It felt so impossible. I was convinced that he would forget me. That he would love them more than me. That he would prefer their care over mine. Their snuggles over mine. Their stories and songs over mine. That the last nine weeks would just disappear. Poof. He wasn't old enough to remember. Obviously the bond from carrying him for nine months and spending each waking (and his sleeping) moment with him would just dissipate.

I had two weekends and one week of solitude with my sweet

babe left. I knew they would be bittersweet. Sweet because they were with him, and I made a promise to myself that I would cherish every single moment. Bitter because each day with him meant one day closer to my inevitable return to work. I tried my best to tell myself that it was going to be okay. To tell myself that I was being unrealistic, dramatic. I prayed endlessly for a door to open that would allow me to stay home. A miracle. I prayed that if that wasn't the plan, for my heart to change. For my heart to be okay with being away from him.

Then, coronavirus.

There had been rumblings. Media had been ramping up with stories about a pandemic and the infamous "two weeks to flatten the curve." Stores and offices were closing to keep people safe. My workplace was notorious for never closing for anything. Living in the Midwest, this included copious amounts of snow. Always open.

And then they decided to close.

It was a Sunday when I got the news. One week from my last day of maternity leave.

They were closing through the end of the month. That was two weeks. I had two more weeks with him. My countdown went from seven days to twenty-one.

I was ecstatic.

I was also terrified.

Despite the fact that no part of me wanted to return to work, I was pushing those emotions down. Or trying to. Out of sight, out of mind, right? Two more weeks meant that I would have to go through this all over again. I would have to feel all of these things again. And they wouldn't be watered-down, second-hand feelings. They were going to be fresh, raw emotions, because I was going to spend two extra weeks watching him grow. He was going to be two weeks older. Two weeks more aware of his surroundings. Two weeks more connected (I hoped) to me.

I was so thankful. And so scared.

Days passed.

Weeks.

Our state issued an extensive stay-at-home order. My work remained closed for business and was expected to remain closed for the foreseeable future, as one of the final industries allowed to reopen.

I was in disbelief. The world was crazy. But this was my miracle. I felt guilty calling it that because it was quite the opposite for so many, but it was. I had prayed for a miracle. This wasn't what I had in mind. But it was giving me precious time with my baby that I could only have dreamed of.

Despite the fact that I knew this would come to an end eventually, I perfected the art of dismissing my emotions regarding work. In my head, I knew that this wasn't good. I was not operating in a healthy way, even though I was truly happy. Joyful, even.

Seventy-four days.

And then it happened. I got the call.

I knew it would be coming at some point. I just didn't expect it when it finally did come. The call that would change everything. I had to go back to work.

I cried. I sobbed, actually. And then I cried a little more.

Work.

Work had become a distant thought again.

In the back of my mind, I knew we wouldn't be forced to stay home forever. That wasn't realistic, even optimistically. I had fallen under the premise that I would have about two weeks to prepare myself between hearing a reopening plan and actually having to be back in the swing of things. Time to mentally and emotionally prepare. Time to get him used to being with someone else during the day. All day . . .

But that wasn't what happened.

The call came on a Thursday afternoon.

I had to be back to work on Monday.

I was wrecked. I couldn't stop crying.

How was I supposed to do this? How was I supposed to go from exclusively being at home with my boy for almost five months to working full-time in THREE DAYS? And it wasn't even going to be normal. It wasn't going to be what I expected to go back to. We were only opening a little bit. Only part of our team was going back. Somehow, I'd drawn the short straw. My failure to understand my role in our reopening made it even harder to wrap my mind around it.

In the time it took for the words to be spoken, the last seventy-four days had vanished. I was right back where I had been, only this time it was worse. Even though I'd anticipated lots of emotions about going back to work, I didn't expect the immensity of what I was feeling. It was like a small panic attack. I felt horrible for my boss. He knew what a blow this was, and he was the one who had to deliver it. And then I bawled like a baby on the phone despite my best efforts.

My soul ached. All of the same feelings came back like a gale wind.

My head KNEW that everything was going to be just fine. He would be safe. He would be happy. He would remember me. It would be good for him to engage with people other than me. It would be good for him to develop relationships with people other than me. I value all of those things, so why did this feel so impossible?

The rest of me couldn't catch up with my head. I felt broken.

And then I made a decision. I had three days left at home with him. There was no way I could just up and quit my job. As much as I regretted it now, this WAS the plan. Inevitable. Impending.

I needed to choose joy.

I needed to embrace every millisecond with him. It wasn't worth my time to sulk. Time had always been precious to me, and now it was rare and beautiful and I needed to make the most of it.

My three days flew by. Faster than I could have imagined. I did my best to process all of my negative emotions rather than stuffing them (yay progress, am I right?). I didn't do a great job of it, but I acknowledged them and their influence on me.

We read. We snuggled (not his favorite, but I'm bigger, so…). We laughed. We sang. We jumped. And jumped some more. And at bedtime, I held him just a little bit longer and a little bit tighter. Somehow, his contentedness calmed me. Reassured me.

I knew he would be okay. I wasn't so sure about me.

The anticipation and anxiety that Sunday night were unreal.

I wanted to just run away. Money and responsibilities would figure themselves out if I wanted it badly enough, right?

I was frustrated.

I was sad.

I was nervous.

I already missed him.

Monday.

I somehow managed to not cry. Not when dropping him off. Not even when driving to work.

It was painful.

I was present for everything that I needed to for work, but all I thought about was him.

Was he okay?

Had he forgotten me already?

Was he sleeping? Eating?

Would he be excited to see me?

Would he want to come home with me?

How many more days did I have to do this?

The answer to that last one wasn't kind.

Every time I started to lower my guard, the tears were ready. I managed to hold it together all day.

I made it back to him. He was one hundred percent okay. He'd had a great day. Played. Eaten. Slept. Was happy.

I was relieved.

I was sad.

I was exhausted from being both.

We went home, and I spent my little bit of time before he had to go to bed just soaking him in. We might be okay. Well, I might be okay. He was definitely going to be okay. I had to remind myself that that was enough.

I did that, on repeat, wondering every morning as I got him ready to leave if maybe, somehow, today could be the last day. I still do that each day. I still don't know the answer. And I'm learning to accept that I may never know. It's not as simple as it seems. I realize that now. I regret that I didn't consider the complexity of how much I would love this little human, and how that would change everything.

My goals.

My passions.

My ambitions.

All that I want is the very best for him. I want him to be happy. I want him to grow up knowing how immensely he is loved. It's still hard for me to accept that I don't have to be at home with him for every second of every day in order for that to happen. I still want that, but it's complicated. Life is complicated. Finances are complicated. Schedules are complicated. Dreams are complicated, even when they're simple.

I find myself trapped. Every fiber of my being wants to be with him every moment. My heart, my soul. But my brain is trying to be logical. It's trying to maintain my realistic optimism, despite my constant heightened emotional state. I want what's best for him. How do I know what's best for him?

We can provide so much more for him if I continue working. He can develop close relationships with family. He can learn to appreciate and respect others. He can learn about more things. He can experience more things. Logically, I know that all of those things will benefit him. I know that they will be conducive to helping build a strong foundation for a caring, well-rounded little boy and young man.

I'm terrified of giving in to that mindset. Not because I don't want that, because that's exactly what I want.

I'm scared of missing anything. Everything. Scared he'll do all of his "first" things when he's not with me. Scared that he'll want me less. Scared that things won't be the way that I expect them to be, regardless of the fact that nothing I want now is what I expected.

And now my mindset that staying home is what I want is giving me doubts, too. Do I really want to stay home? Or is this just an adjustment that I have to make? Is this a quality vs. quantity thing? Will our time together be more special if I'm working? Will it not? Would we actually be able to make it if I wasn't working full-time?

I don't know which sacrifices I'm willing to make. Maybe that's the hardest part. It's also the part that scares and saddens me the most.

So I remind myself of what I KNOW to be true.

Wanting to stay at home does not make you a bad wife. Wanting to go to work does not make you a bad mama.

Let me rephrase that. And repeat it, over and over again.

Wanting to stay at home does not make me a bad wife.

Wanting to go to work does not make me a bad mama.

So I wait.

I wait for clarity.

I wait for a door to open.

A window.

A vent.

Anything.

I wait for another miracle.

I celebrate the time that I do have with him, every moment. I celebrate the extra seventy-seven days that I had to spend with him.

They were a gift. I realize now how immense of a gift.

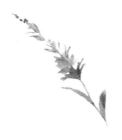

the after

Me.

I.

I don't know who "me" is anymore. And I'm struggling with that. I don't know if the "me" that existed before our baby boy is here. I don't know if it's possible for her to exist. Or if I want her to exist.

I'm stuck in this indeterminate state of Mama. I LOVE being Mama. It's like he is everything that life was missing, and I just didn't know it until he arrived.

I find so much joy in being Mama.

So much gratitude.

So much challenging fulfillment.

Becoming Mama changed me. It changed me in ways that I didn't know needed to be changed. It transformed all of my desires and aspirations. It strengthened my convictions. It has grown me.

But somewhere in the midst of becoming, I lost me.

I guess when you're focused on learning how to keep a little human alive, that makes sense.

He came first during my desperate grasping for stable ground amidst my postpartum journey. But then even after I found a rhythm, he still comes first. My husband, too, but never me.

And I'm not trying to make this sound like a pity party for myself. It's NOT. I literally don't know how to do that.

But I miss me.

I miss having a sense of self outside of Mama.

I miss feeling like I have everything together.

I miss feeling as though I'm succeeding as a wife.

I miss feeling as though I'm succeeding as ME.

I feel guilty for even saying that because it feels like I'm giving some admission of wrong. Like I'm saying that I don't love my baby enough. Like I'm saying that I don't WANT to be Mama.

That is the furthest thing from the truth, but I'm struggling to find a balance of them. HOW to be Mama, and Wife, and still find the time and energy to be me. And to figure out who that is anymore.

Or is it enough, what I DO know?

I love Jesus.

I love my husband.

I love being his wife.

I love my son.

I love being Mama.

I love rainstorms and fall weather.

I love decorating for Christmas and listening to Christmas music long before it's considered socially acceptable.

I love coffee.

I love the woods and the mountains.

I love making deep connections with others, especially those who take the time to care for me as much as I do for them.

I love helping others feel empowered and valued and loved.

Folgers commercials still make me cry.

It feels like there should be more, like I should be more complex than that.

I should BE more. DO more.

I find myself in what feels like an identity crisis. Before going back to work, I sobbed at the idea of leaving him every day. I learned to turn my emotions off at work so that I wouldn't sob there. Days turned into weeks, weeks into months, and everything started changing.

Some days I've loved being a big girl and using my brain and having real, adult things to be responsible for (as if a baby weren't).

Some days I've wanted to curl up in a ball with the little guy and never leave the house again.

Some days I still love being a big girl.

Some days I still want to cry in the corner and snuggle my babe.

Some days I feel proud.

Some days I feel guilty.

Most days I feel guilty.

I've realized that this isn't going to change. I wish I could say that there was a moment where everything shifted for me, that at some spontaneous time, all of my ambitions and emotions returned to what I thought would be normal.

It's really just not going to happen.

Maybe it will for you. It might. But I pray that it doesn't.

I pray that you continue to grow and change. That you continue to bloom.

It is becoming more and more apparent to me just how important this part of the journey is.

No matter where you are in your journey, have courage, dear heart. People aren't joking when they say that being a parent isn't easy. Unfortunately, that's usually as far as the conversation goes and you're stuck, not knowing what to expect.

The truth? Expect nothing, and expect everything. Each and every moment is going to change you. You won't recognize yourself for a while, and you shouldn't. Carrying and bringing a sweet babe into the world, and the life that comes after, is world-changing. You will not be the same. Remember that that is okay. You're allowed to feel. You're allowed to change what you think that you want. You will start to think in ways that you've never thought before and in ways that you never expected to. Little decisions become huge considerations, and things that used to be so important, they just don't even hold a light to this sweet little person that you've created.

And every one of those things is OKAY.

You are allowed to change.

You are allowed to feel.

You are allowed to allow yourself to do those things.

So, to everyone who told me during pregnancy to "just wait" for those things that seemed so daunting and negative . . . I'm still waiting.

Waiting for this to be as bad as you made it sound like it might be.

Waiting to be unpleasantly surprised.

Waiting to . . . I don't even know what. Have a regret? Say you were right?

Because beyond all of those big feelings, I just can't find anything but love, joy, and gratitude.

Even on our WORST day—and trust me, we are so far from perfect—I cannot imagine life without this little boy.

Have things changed? YES.

Are there challenges? Absolutely.

Do I know what I'm doing? Not a clue.

But I know that I was made to bring him into this world and be exactly the mama that he needs. We can figure out the rest, together.

So, I'll keep waiting. Not expecting anything. But sowing all of the reward.

I believe that we are CHOSEN to be mothers to the children that we have, so if you are struggling with worthiness, please don't. You were made to be everything that sweet babe needs. You already have it in you. That means that you are enough. You are adequate. You are sufficient. You CAN do this. It won't always feel like it, but you can, and you will, because every time those big, beautiful eyes look up at you, you'll know. You're right where you belong.

. . . .

Like I said, this is just my story. I pray that it will meet you where you are and give you whatever you're looking for.

A new perspective.

A laugh.

Validation.

Hope.

I pray that your people will love you hard and that you'll allow them to.

I pray that you'll be brave and ask for the help that you need when you need it.

I pray that you will remember that you are worthy, and capable, and STRONG.

I pray that you will remember that just as your sweet babe was created inside of you, so you were created for them.

To be Mama.

Their Mama.

And, if you forget these things, I pray that you will allow yourself to remember, so that you can bloom into the Mama that you were created to be, too.

In case no one has told you, I'm proud of you.

I'm proud of the work that you're doing.

I'm proud that you care enough to do everything in your power to give that sweet babe of yours everything that they need. I'm proud that you care enough to do everything in your power to give yourself everything that you need.

If you need more support, if you need to vent, or if you just need to hear from someone else that YOU CAN DO THIS, shoot me an email. I'd love to chat.

kyleefrederick@proton.me

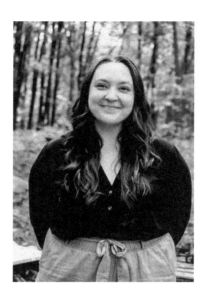

Hi! I'm Kylee—a creative, authentic old soul who believes in finding beauty in the chaos and using my gifts to serve and empower others. (un)expecting is my first book—the first of many tools I hope to offer to mamas who were/are (or aren't) struggling as much as I did. Before dedicating my life to my tiny human, I received an undergraduate degree in Addictions Counseling and Psychology—and then ended up working in Early Childhood and Health & Wellness instead. I live in the Mitten (Michigan) with my husband and son and love every moment that life offers us. Any free time is spent writing, crafting, baking, making music, watching BBC shows and action movies, or being outside in this beautiful world God created. Thanks for joining me on this journey to better love and serve one another.

CPSIA information can be obtained
at www.ICGtesting.com
Printed in the USA
BVHW092321131022
649416BV00007B/35

9 781645 384724